25 months

by

Beth and
Jason Brubaker

Stock photo images by Shutterstock

Printed in the United States of America

First Printing, 2023

ISBN 978-1-955791-76-2

Library of Congress Control Number: 2023919074

Ordering Information: Special discounts are available on quantity purchases by bookstores, corporations, associations, and others. For details, contact the publisher at sales@braughlerbooks.com or at 937-58-BOOKS.

For questions or comments about this book, please write to Info@braughlerbooks.com.

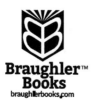

Braughler™
Books
braughlerbooks.com

FOREWORD

May 21, 2020

Dear Harper,

Happy birthday, sweet girl. Dada and I love you so much.

This year has been the best of our lives. Even with all the sleepless nights, endless number of diapers, and a lot of spit up, we had first snuggles, first (and a million) laughs, first steps, and first "dadas" and kind of "mamas." Our hearts grew by a million because of what you have brought to our family.

Harper, I wish I could say that everything was easy over the last two years. That's really where this started - 25 months ago, to be exact. We prayed for you for months and months and worried you would never join our family. Then, in the midst of the greatest storm of our lives, God brought a rainbow. He brought us you. His timing is always perfect, and having you with us during every doctor's appointment, every surgery, and every chemotherapy treatment gave us hope for the incredible future that God was creating for us.

About six months ago, we realized that your first birthday and my last treatment would fall on the same day. I cried. It was the perfect ending to an unbelievable story. It is an ending that only God could have written for us. Like everything we have been through in the past two years, God's fingerprints were all over it.

< 1 >

Today, we celebrated you - our forever smiling, happy, strawberry blonde spitfire - whose improbable, yet perfectly timed, entrance got both of us through the absolute worst moments of our lives. You are a constant reminder to us that miracles happen. You were possible but improbable, given the circumstances. However, as we know, God does not make mistakes, and you were very much supposed to be here on this journey with me. I am convinced that the experience of being pregnant and a new mom while going through treatment is the reason that I emotionally and physically handled it all far better than expected. You continue to give us something in which to look forward.

Today, we celebrated the end of a defining chapter of our lives - the end of your first year and the end of my time as a cancer patient. Tonight, surrounded by our family and close friends (via Zoom), we watched you devour cake by the fistful for the first time... and love it. Today, surrounded by the incredible doctors, nurses, and medical staff who have become members of our extended family, the beeping of the IV machine at Cancer Care went off for the last time as my final treatment bags ran empty. So many tears and socially distanced/virtual hugs (such an odd time we live in).

Harper, this is the close of one chapter and the start of so much more. Because of modern medicine, our incredible tribe of family and friends, and faith in a God who is a good father, I will be able to walk with you through the coming mountains and valleys. I am so grateful for the opportunity.

I love you so much. Thank you for being my daughter.

Love,
Mama

< 2 >

1. MISCARRIAGE

Beth: Did you know that you only have a 20% chance of getting pregnant each month? You have a week of pre-fertility and then 1-2 days that "it happens." It seems so easy when you are not in the throes of it.

Jason and I were together for almost six years prior to getting married. After getting married, we decided we would begin the process of starting a family. We checked all of the boxes first:

Got married. Check.

Sold a house. Check.

Bought a bigger house. Check.

We were ready.

In the fall of 2017, we started trying. It was a little concerning at the beginning because of our ages (31 and 35) and others around us had struggled… plus, neither of us is known for our patience.

Month after month, nothing. We began to get a little bit worried.

Then, in March 2018, after Jason and I celebrated our 1-year wedding anniversary (and a lot of wine at "The Melting Pot"), I took a pregnancy test after work.

< 3 >

Blue cross. I was pregnant.

I ran to Walmart and bought the cutest monkey socks and a gift bag. I hid that and the pregnancy test in a laundry basket, hoping to surprise Jason, but then right before he got home, I couldn't find it.

So I just told him and cried - a running theme in this story.

We called our families and shared more tears. I remember sending my sister-in-law (who was also pregnant with our nephew, Griffin) a picture of a shirt that said "Big Cousin" while she was at the park. She called, crying, and we talked about how Griffin and our little one would only be six months apart.

We were bursting with joy and excitement in our house. I took pictures in the mirror to see if my stomach looked bigger. We were overjoyed.

We stayed busy. Over spring break, the baby and I joined some of my colleagues in a protest in Frankfort against Governor Matt Bevin related to proposed teacher pension reform. We also told our closest friends the good news and did what we could to prepare for what was to come. We scheduled doctors' appointments, got all the paperwork through the OB's office, and were just generally excited.

Until three weeks later. Blood. Spotting at school.

I called the nurse line.

"Spotting is normal - happens in about 30% of pregnancies," she reassured me. "Everything is fine."

Until it got worse.

< 4 >

Jason: *I will freely admit that I had not given a whole lot of thought to miscarriages for most of my life. Naturally, I knew they occurred, but I just didn't have much context around the subject. I would hear about somebody getting pregnant and I would just expect that in about nine months, they'd have a baby. That's how it is supposed to work.*

It wasn't until it hit people close to me that I even really learned much about them, and why they occurred, and how painful it was. Witnessing people you care about go through a miscarriage is terrible. There's nothing you can really say, no actions you can take, to make it better. You feel helpless.

> **Beth:** The nurse scheduled me for an ultrasound, and the ultrasound technician (who I came to love) showed us a heartbeat at 134 beats per minute.
>
> A heartbeat. A little slow, but not a concern. We exhaled and cried. Everything you read is that after hearing a heartbeat, the chance of miscarriage drops significantly — from 25% to 5%.

I wasn't concerned until she asked me when my last period was. I told her, and she paused.

"Are you sure?"

> The technician mentioned the baby was measuring about a week behind, but "that happens." We rejoiced.

She advised pelvic rest and sent us on our way.

> Two nights later, around 4 am, I began to bleed — huge clots. I was starting to miscarry. I remember saying to Jason that something was wrong. This wasn't normal. I was cramping terribly.

< 5 >

During the school day, I called the doctor's office and they scheduled another ultrasound. They continued to tell me that all was fine.

Jason: *For a couple days after we first heard a heartbeat, Beth had been spotting and was understandably worried. I was less so, mainly because I was just ignorant. Like with many things that would happen to us over the coming months, I was just in way over my head in terms of grasping the situation. I didn't know what was or wasn't supposed to be happening at this point. How could I?*

> *Besides, we had just heard the heartbeat. Everything was fine. I agreed to meet her at the doctor's office that afternoon, but the thought that something might really be wrong hadn't yet sunk into my mind.*

> **Beth:** I went to the ultrasound alone. Jason was stuck in traffic. I went in and had a different ultrasound tech this time. I saw the sac and the baby.

"There is no heartbeat."

Jason: *I was in my car, about 10-15 minutes from the hospital when Beth called. Her first words were "There's no heartbeat."*

It took a few seconds for my brain to process that, followed by a stream of jumbled thoughts that I couldn't quite turn into words.

No heartbeat? Tell them to do something. We just heard it! They must be wrong. Tell them to check again!!

> **Beth:** It's hard for me to remember the moments immediately after. I remember sitting in a hallway between the ultrasound room and the doctor's office waiting for Jason. I am not sure how long it actually took, but it felt like an eternity. People passed me in the hallway and saw me crying.

< 6 >

Jason: *I covered the last eight miles of the drive in about five minutes. I rushed from my car into the hospital and punched the elevator button furiously. Of all the places to have a slow elevator, the hospital felt especially cruel. I finally got to the second floor, turned right out of the elevator and saw Beth walking toward me, tears running down her face.*

We may or may not have said anything in that moment; I honestly don't remember. It started to become a blur right about then.

They took us to an office where a nurse talked to us for a few minutes, and then taken to meet a doctor in his office. He explained what had happened and also explained, from a medical standpoint, what the next steps would be. I was listening, hearing him speak, but most of it wasn't processing. It seemed too sudden. A few days ago, we heard our baby's heartbeat. Now we didn't have a baby? How could that be? How could everything change so quickly?

Beth: There is nothing quite like sitting in a doctor's office after a miscarriage. What I appreciated so much that day was the doctor on call. He was one of my favorite OBs in the practice because of his dry sense of humor. There is nothing quite like it.

However, in that moment, his tone was somber. He said to us, "You are allowed to be sad right now. You lost a child."

A child. You are not supposed to lose a child. Yesterday, I was pregnant, and today, I am not.

The doctor scheduled a D and C for the next day with one of his colleagues, whom he said was one of the best.

He told us that "it was not my fault" and "this was not uncommon," adding it was likely a chromosomal defect.

With a heavy sigh, he said, "unfortunately, these things just happen."

Jason: *As we left the hospital, the numbness continued to set it. I remember texting my parents with the news but saying that we didn't really want to talk right now. I remember getting in my car and then I remember pulling into our driveway. Nothing in between. It was like a fog had set over my mind, where I was only able to intermittently break through it to recognize what I was doing in that moment.*

> *Once home, we didn't say much. We sat in our front room, wiping away tears and feeling very alone, despite the fact that we were sitting right next to each other.*

> **Beth:** I have never felt that sense of loss in my entire life. We went home, and without going into the details, I passed the pregnancy at home in our bathroom. It was the most intense physical pain I had ever had, and the most horrific emotional pain of my life. I ended up being hospitalized overnight to make sure that I would not need surgery in the morning.

Jason: *Around 9:00 that night, about six hours after the news that had irreparably changed our lives, I stepped out of our hospital room into the hallway to call my parents and let them know we would be staying the night.*

My dad answered and I got maybe three words out before the tears came. It turns out that saying the words out loud was almost as painful as hearing them. I ducked into a corner, away from the nurses' desk, where I just let the tears come. It could have been 10 seconds or 10 minutes – I wasn't sure. But I believe it was in that moment that I really grasped what had happened and how much it hurt.

I also recognized in that moment that this was going to leave a permanent scar.

We had lost a child. We had a child and then we didn't. There is no way to explain the pain you feel from that, even though we never met him. And there is no

< 8 >

way people who haven't been through it can fully understand why it hurts so much. It's a pain I wouldn't wish on my worst enemy.

Beth: I remember looking at the ultrasound screen and seeing nothing.

No more heartbeat.

No more sac.

No more baby.

Jason: *We would return to our house the next morning, where we both crashed. To say we were drained would be an understatement. Emotionally, mentally, physically...we had nothing left. I don't recall ever feeling so exhausted. It was a bright, sunny, April day and all we both wanted to do was shut the world out and be alone.*

We closed the blinds, locked the doors, turned off our phones. Outside, the world went on as it normally would on a spring Friday. But inside, our world was forever changed and we just weren't sure how to begin accepting that.

Beth: April 19, 2018. The day our son died. I thought from the moment I became pregnant that it was a boy. Even though we cannot be sure... I am sure. We are sure.

Jason: *In one way, that weekend brought us closer together than maybe we'd ever been. We both were experiencing it differently, but we were experiencing it together. There were a lot of unspoken words that weekend, but that was okay. We both just knew what the other was thinking and feeling. It was perhaps the one bright spot over the next few weeks — that connection we had established through a shared tragedy.*

< 9 >

A few days later, we ended up planting a rose bush in our backyard in memory of our son. As we prayed over it, holding back tears, I remember thinking this was, without a doubt, the hardest thing I had ever gone through.

There was no way we could have known, in that moment, that our journey was getting ready to get a whole lot harder.

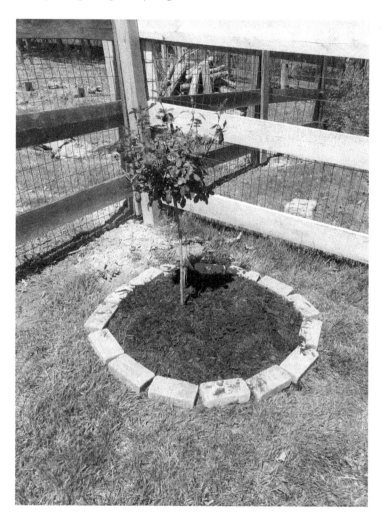

< 10 >

2. GRIFFIN

Jason: *The next couple of weeks seemed to drag on as we tried to resume some sense of normalcy, even though it was never far from our minds. Instead of getting a nursery ready or loading up on diapers, we were still coming to grips with what happened. We didn't mention it out loud often, but it was always there.*

But all of that was put on hold about three weeks later as we prepared for my second nephew to arrive. Though my sister was being induced early, she and my brother-in-law seemed calm and composed at the hospital. No panic or worry that something might go wrong.

After days and days of tears, it was refreshing to be surrounded by a sense of hope again. Our family was growing and we were ready to welcome a beautiful baby boy to this world. It didn't make our pain disappear, but it helped it subside, even if just for a few hours in the hospital as we waited.

Beth: There is truly nothing like being an aunt. It's all the perks of being a mom while still being able to give the screaming child back to their parents. Harrison, our first nephew, brought us an incredible amount of joy. We were so fortunate to be able to see him at least once a month during his first year. Harrison waddled down the aisle at our wedding as the honorary ring bearer, only just learning to walk.

< 11 >

When we found out we were pregnant, one of the first thoughts I had was that our family would welcome two miracles in the same year. You can't help but to begin planning the months to come.

And then the miscarriage.

Jason: *Whenever a painful thought entered my mind, like wondering if we would ever find ourselves in the hospital awaiting the birth of our child, I did my best to suppress it. This day wasn't about us, and I tried to put on that brave face as best as I could, even if being in a hospital again was giving me some anxiety.*

Beth: Shortly after Griffin arrived late that Friday afternoon, he was taken to the NICU for observation for his lungs. His heart, thankfully, was just fine. We celebrated with cookies and hugs, and like before, everything seemed fine.

Jason: *Griffin's arrival late on Friday afternoon was joyous, as it should be. Though we knew he would have to spend some time in the NICU for the development of his lungs, the general consensus seemed pretty positive at first.*

Beth: Going to that hospital to see Griffin is one of the hardest things I have ever done. Even now, I feel so guilty saying that. I cried the entire two-hour ride to Lexington. Honestly, I had contemplated not coming at all. The idea of seeing babies absolutely ravaged my soul. It felt like the cruelest joke imaginable. We had just lost our son, and now, we had to go to a place where there were the most tangible reminders of the baby we would never get to bring home.

< 12 >

Fortunately, our family understood. My mother-in-law, one of my favorite people on the planet, asked if I needed some air. It was like she knew I felt like I was drowning.

She took me outside to a really pretty garden in front of the hospital. She sat on a bench with me, and her words were what I needed to hear.

"You are so brave for being here. I don't know if I could have come."

It was like she read my mind. It had been three weeks, and although I physically was back to normal, I felt like I had been crushed from the inside out. I told her the same thing I told Jason and anyone else who asked.

"I wasn't missing this moment. I would have regretted it forever."

What either of us didn't realize was things were about to turn very quickly.

After an hour or so, we had the opportunity to see Griffin in the NICU. When Harrison was born, the NICU was under construction, so the poor guy was in his incubator in a tiny room with three other babies. Now, we entered a spacious, brightly colored yellow hallway to sanitize prior to going back.

As we waited for the doors to open, it was hard to keep it together. I could feel hot tears dripping down my face and quickly tried to wipe them with my sleeve. I felt so guilty in worrying about how my feelings as opposed to that little boy. I didn't want anyone to see me cry, especially my sister-in-law. She has become a sister to me, and it is a relationship that I am so grateful for... she was the one I was most nervous to impress when Jason and I started dating. A sister's opinion is important... just ask my brother.

Jason came over to me and kept asking if I was okay.

< 13 >

More loudly than I realized, I said, "Yes. STOP."

Everyone looked at me for a brief moment - a nanosecond.

However, that was long enough. Everyone noticed.

I could feel my face turn beet red. How selfish could I be? Our nephew was in the NICU, and my concern was my feelings - my broken heart. I sanitized my hands and walked in.

For a place where babies are sick, the NICU, on its exterior, is a beautiful place. It is brightly colored - greens and yellows. It had been renovated since Harrison was born. The night he was born - he was in a little room crammed with incubators. Griffin, instead, had his own space.

We walked into the room - it was spacious but sparse. Just the incubator, equipment, and a cot. Griffin, by all accounts, looked good. He had issues with oxygen, but that was typical for a 36-weeker. Nurses came in and out, but again, he looked okay.

Jason: *Seeing Griffin that day brought a flood of emotions. Adding to those was the fact that he was hooked up to a number of machines and had wires seemingly running everywhere. I blinked back a tear as we walked into the room.*

Even in the best of circumstances, seeing a little baby, helpless, hooked into enormous machines with wires and lights and beeping sounds...it's tough. He didn't deserve this. He didn't deserve to start his life this way. He was an innocent baby, just a couple hours old. My sister and brother-in-law are strong people, incredibly strong, and I remember wondering just how they were managing to keep it together so well.

< 14 >

Beth: Looking back, I am grateful and thankful that I had enough sense to go see him. It was Mother's Day weekend. We said our goodbyes and headed back to Cincinnati.

That Sunday, Mother's Day, I sat on our front porch - we are fortunate to have an amazing covered front porch. It's one of my favorite places to sit. I texted Stacie - "Happy Mother's Day - what a wonderful way to celebrate."

About an hour later, we realized how inappropriate that text was.

We got a phone call from Jason's mom. Griffin had been transferred to the University of Kentucky Medical Center. It was a life-or-death situation. Griffin had stopped breathing and needed immediate intervention. As it was described to us, they literally ran with Griffin into the ambulance and then ran with him into the hospital. Jason's mom said she would call with more information after a surgery to place Griffin on an ECMO machine.

Jason: *We were told that, for a number of reasons, his chances of survival were not high. Getting that phone call early on Sunday morning with that news was almost unbearable. We had been through so much as a family already....why was this happening? My body went numb, just like it had a few weeks earlier.*

Beth: The hope would be that this machine would work as an artificial lung to allow Griffin's lungs to heal. Jason could not sit still for an instant. He was restless. Jason is not one to show emotion on his sleeve (unlike his wife). However, in that instant, his face turned ghostly white.

Jason: *We wanted to jump in the car and head down to Lexington right away, but it was decided that it was better for us to hold off. There was*

< 15 >

enough going on and we didn't want to add to the chaos. However, I did volunteer to call several other family members with the news.

Beth, who knows me better than I like to let on, asked if I was up for that and I foolishly told her I was. I walked out to our front porch to call our great-uncle, who kind of serves as the unofficial patriarch of my dad's side of the family.

Just like the call I made from the hospital three weeks earlier, I couldn't get even one full sentence out before I started choking up. Beth stepped outside and grabbed the phone from my hands, delivering the news that I couldn't even find a way to vocalize through tears.

Beth: I took the phone and explained what was happening. Jason was right - saying the words made it real.

After finishing the conversation, I looked at Jason, who was already at his feet.

"I need to move."

So we did. We walked around the neighborhood... just the two of us. Waiting for another phone call. There was an estimated time, but we hadn't heard anything.

Jason: I can honestly say that was the longest afternoon of my life as we waited for that phone call. We prayed and talked and tried to stay positive, but trying to relieve that anxiety was a fruitless effort. At some point, I began mentally preparing myself for bad news, perhaps just to steady myself if that's what was to come.

< 16 >

We finally received a call from my mom late that afternoon - the surgery had gone well and Griffin was now resting. He still had a long road ahead of him, but he had already shown he was a fighter.

We didn't know a lot of the other details that day, such as the next steps for Griffin, or how long he had to stay in the hospital. Plenty more answers would come in the following days and weeks. The fear and sadness and grief was all still very real. But he was alive.

Beth: Griffin did more than survive - he is a fun, intelligent, and adventurous kindergartner now. He truly reminded us that God works miracles beyond our understanding. We would need that reminder again and again.

< 17 >

< 18 >

3. GRIEF

Jason: *As spring turned to summer, things slowly started to begin to go back to normal, at least outwardly. We enjoyed grilling out, playing in the yard with our dogs, walking up the street to get ice cream in the evenings. Anyone observing us would have never guessed what was going on internally with each of us.*

Beth: One of the best parts of our marriage is that we keep things pretty light-hearted in our house. What I mean by WE is Jason. Jason keeps us grounded and laughing all of the time. There are few evenings that we do not laugh about something.

However, this was different.

There was silence in our house.

No laughing.

No joy.

Just deafening silence.

There was before the miscarriage and after.

We were both shells of ourselves. We went through the paces of our normal routines. Jason went to work every day, and because of the summer break, I

< 19 >

did things around the house. We ate dinner together. We watched TV and spent time together.

But something was missing. A void that felt like it would never be filled.

Jason: *Grieving is such an interesting phenomenon. There's tons and tons of research and literature on the grieving process and how to help people cope with grief. And I don't discount any of that. But when you get down to it, everyone grieves differently because everyone feels and thinks differently. That's just a fact of life and I think everyone, on some level, recognizes that.*

Yet for whatever reason, we struggled to reconcile that with each other, with our grieving processes occasionally manifesting into resentment, anger, sadness and hopelessness. There were times we became divided, rather than standing shoulder to shoulder to face the grief together.

Beth: Jason and I tend to approach things differently. Jason is a far more logical thinker than I am. I tend to lead with my emotions. We offset each other very well.

Those differences, though, were amplified more so than ever before. We were both suffering such a tremendous loss, but it was like we could not understand the process of grief that the other was going through. We were not speaking the same language.

We fought. A LOT. We said so many terrible things to one another. Our loss, instead of bringing us together, was ripping us apart. We just could not get back in sync.

Jason: *I tried to compartmentalize my emotions to avoid letting them control every waking moment. Because the sad reality is that the world doesn't stop spinning when something tragic happens to you. You still*

< 20 >

have to go to work and there are still bills that need to be paid. You still need to wash dishes, mow the yard, feed the dogs, take the trash out, fold laundry, buy groceries, and do the million other things that are just part of our routines.

And so by continuing to do these things, I wasn't trying to bury or hide my grief; I simply was recognizing that these things still need to happen. Maybe I would take a private moment to myself on the drive to work, or grapple with some tough thoughts as I pushed the lawnmower around, but I did my best to not let the hurt inside stop me from living life and doing what needs to be done. Right or wrong, that's just how I am.

Beth, on the other hand, has always worn her heart on her sleeve. There's no hiding how she feels. Plus, there's also no denying that even though we say that we had a miscarriage, the reality is that she physically experienced it, which is obviously entirely different. And though I tried to be sympathetic, that was just a reality I couldn't ever understand because I hadn't physically experienced it. Though we were both in the same situation of having lost a baby, we were experiencing it from two entirely different points of view.

And it was miserable for both of us. We were both hurting and taking it out on each other.

Beth: My trip to Salt Lake City could not have come at a better time. For the previous three years, I traveled to Utah in June to score Advanced Placement tests for the subject area I teach. I thoroughly enjoy learning how to be a better teacher and seeing my colleagues and friends for two weeks each year. There is an "OG" group who read and muddled through

< 21 >

teaching the course since 2014. We always enjoyed everything SLC has to offer - urban hiking, fantastic food and beer, and a beautiful location.

Like every June, Jason dropped me at the airport and gave me an enormous hug and kiss. I looked at him and started crying. At that moment, I did not want to leave. I did not want to have to see my friends. I did not want to have to explain why I looked bloated and a little pudgy.

This was supposed to be the trip where I was able to share with my friends that Jason and I were finally pregnant.

Instead, I sat in the terminal, crying over my bagel. It just was not fair.

Jason: *In normal circumstances, I didn't mind Beth going away for a couple of weeks. The money was good, she got to see a beautiful part of the country, and I got to live a bachelor's existence for a couple weeks (i.e., pizza for dinner basically every night). We talked every day, but it was nice to get a little time for ourselves too.*

But this year, it just felt different. It was different. The chasm that had existed between us for a few weeks felt like it was growing larger with her trip. It was hard to pinpoint an exact feeling but everything just felt... unsettled. Incomplete.

Beth: For the reading this year, there were two waves of people arriving. I was part of the "late-arriving" table leader group. My roommate for the previous year had already been there for a week. She is from Alabama, and actually teaches a different AP subject, but that subject fits well with mine. She has the most amazing accent and always reminded me of southern hospitality. Seeing her made the anxiety of being away from home immediately leave.

< 22 >

At the AP Reading, we spend long days in a windowless room inside of "The Salt Palace," the convention center for Salt Lake City. We prepare to train teachers how to score the four portions of the exam accurately. We eat the best snacks every few hours. Then, in the evenings, we go to dinner, hike, and more.

It was truly a blessing to be there, but my roommate noticed that something was not right.

One of the first evenings I was there, she finally asked if I was okay.

Like a floodgate, I broke down. I told her everything. I told her I was less than eight weeks out from having a miscarriage, that Griffin had almost died, and that I was struggling with immense guilt and depression. We just sat and talked before going to bed. She told me she knew so many women who had gone through what I was going through. Many of them went on to have healthy pregnancies following the miscarriage.

That moment changed the feelings surrounding the trip. I began to enjoy myself and the people whom I never see. I enjoyed morning walks to the Utah State Capitol and many hikes. We even ventured to Park City for a fancy girls' dinner.

One night, our group went for a hike to Ensign Peak. At the top of this mountain, you have a panoramic view of Salt Lake City and the Great Salt Lake. It is spectacular, especially at the golden hour.

As we snapped our yearly picture together, I stood there, just sad. This should have been the baby's first big trip, baby's first hike, and probably a baby bump (at this point, I would have been 14 weeks).

< 23 >

When our friend showed the picture, I almost broke down right then. You could see a pooch in my stomach where I had tied my sweatshirt. That pooch should have been our son. I could never predict when the grief was going to come.

When we came back from the hike, I went into the bathroom and noticed that a sore on my left nipple that I had for a few months was sticking to the inside of my bra. I saw liquid.

That scared me.

My annual appointment with my OB/GYN was already scheduled to talk about beginning to try again for a baby. It was something that I tucked in the back of my mind to speak to her about.

That year, we finished reading over 30,000 exams and did our closing party at a dueling piano bar. The trip was much needed. We talked about the year after and seeing each other then.

That break is truly what Jason and I needed. Time to sort our feelings.

Jason: *Ultimately, the time apart was probably good, though the lingering feelings were still there. A few weeks ago, we had a baby on the way. Now, I never felt further away from being a parent.*

And the question that neither one of us was ready to truly confront was still there, still lurking in our minds....what if this never happens for us? What if it's just not meant to be?

Beth: The next week brought my annual appointment to the OB/GYN, and I had a list of questions to ask, including about my left nipple.

< 24 >

The OB/GYN ended up running almost an hour behind. When she came in, we talked about starting to try again and if it was safe to do so.

It was. I was so excited that I almost forgot to ask about my left breast.

She told me that nipples have discharge, especially after a miscarriage because of the hormones. If it is clear, it is okay. She also said to call if there was still an issue in a few months.

We filled the next few weeks with an attempt to have a little bit of fun. For my birthday, Jason bought tickets to a Cincinnati Reds game honoring Fiona the Hippo. For attending the game, the Reds were giving out a Fiona bobblehead. Fiona was the premature hippo born at the Cincinnati Zoo on January 24, 2017 (four days before my birthday), and I have a slight obsession with her.

Jason: *It was a perfect night to be at the ballpark and it felt nice to just be out again, having a good time, feeling somewhat normal. Of course, we had no idea what was coming down the road for us, or how much Fiona would actually become part of our story. For that night, we were just two average people, enjoying a carefree baseball game.*

Beth: That night was the first date that Jason and I had been on since losing our son. We had a blast. The Reds won with multiple home runs. We needed that time together.

The month ended with a week-long trip to Chattanooga with a colleague for training in another AP course. I would not teach it, but it was still amazing information. We went hiking and went to a minor-league baseball game.

< 25 >

Another opportunity to forget the immense amount of grief I was feeling.

Jason and I geared up slowly for July… to try again to complete our family. I had my app ready and ovulation tests in hand. We kept telling ourselves we were ready.

We could do this.

< 26 >

4. TRYING AGAIN

Jason: *Physically, emotionally, mentally...we both said we were ready but there were still plenty of doubts.*

What if we got pregnant again, only to suffer another miscarriage?

What if we got pregnant and there was something wrong with the baby?

What if we couldn't get pregnant again?

Beth: After my OB/GYN gave us the green light to begin trying again, the initial excitement melted into fear.

I'll be really frank. The magic of intimacy was gone.

Part of me wanted to give up and not go any further. Our miscarriage may have been God's way of saying that we were not meant to be parents. I was hopeful that this was not true, but why would God let something like this happen?

Jason: *I abhor playing the "what if" game but in this situation, it was almost impossible not to. Because, as obvious as it seems, this was potentially life-changing.*

< 27 >

Having a child or not having a child is two entirely different paths in life, and it felt like we were standing at the proverbial fork-in-the-road, only we didn't really have a choice which way we were going to go.

Beth: Even through this trauma, we continued to live our lives. July and August were absolute blurs. They always are - trying to fit every fun moment of summer while balancing the impending school year stress that always happens prior to the first day.

We hosted our first Fourth of July gathering in our new home, attended a version of "Midsummer's Night Dream" along the Ohio River, and went back to the Melting Pot with our two friends who introduced us.

But there was always the elephant in the room.

When would we actually try again?

We decided that in July... we would. I bought the ovulation tests to control as much as I could... even though we had absolutely no control over this.

Then the two week wait, as it is (not so) affectionately called by anyone who is trying to get pregnant. I bought a cheap pregnancy test from the dollar store on the designated day.

Peed on the stick.

Not pregnant.

Jason: *It was more than a little nerve-wracking. You didn't want to get too excited or think too much about all the fun parts of being a parent. Saturday morning cartoons, Halloween costumes, leaving out cookies for Santa, learning to ride a bike, family vacations to Disney World....all of that.*

< 28 >

Being able to see how a child sees the world, how they grow and develop. That was what we both wanted more than anything. But after having that taken from us earlier, we were anxious. Fearful. Maybe even a little cynical. We wondered if perhaps we were being punished for something.

Beth: It was like feeling the emptiness of the miscarriage all over again. If there had not been a miscarriage, I would be five months pregnant. We would not be doing this again.

Trauma comes in waves. Grief comes in waves.

Again, we were grieving the child we never met.

Jason: *Outwardly, I remained positive. But the doubt was growing. Maybe this just wasn't meant to be for us.*

I tried to find silver linings, even if just in my own thinking, to rationalize it all. No question that not having a baby provided us with more freedom in our daily lives. It definitely left more money in our pockets. And who really wants to change dirty diapers anyway?

But deep down, I knew I was just trying to mask my grief and frustration. It left me feeling hollow.

Beth: August brought prepping for the upcoming school year. This year, I was asked to finally teach Journalism — my true love - after a seven-year hiatus. I met with my new Journalism student editors and yearbook representative to plan. I decorated my classroom in bright yellows complete with inspirational quotes.

I promised myself that this would be my school year.

< 29 >

I was teaching exactly what I wanted to.

We had a new principal who wanted to integrate fun into our school culture.

Everything seemed to be coming together.

> The weeks before school brought some fun moments. Two colleagues and I traveled to Indianapolis to see Walk The Moon, one of my favorite bands. I also saw two of my sorority sisters for a margarita and a reminiscing session after not seeing them in several years.

> My first day of school involved hype up music, running into an auditorium with students cheering, helping with service projects, meeting my first journalism class in seven years, and handing out 1,300 teacher appreciation cards to our teachers districtwide.

It was going to be an incredible school year.

> But in the midst of things going well professionally, the four walls of our house felt empty. We had hoped that our first month of actual "trying" would have brought us some light.

Nothing.

Now August.

Nothing.

> The hopelessness we both felt was evident. I asked Jason so many times the same question.

"What if this is never going to happen for us?"

< 30 >

Jason: *It was tough. We both had tons of friends who had gotten pregnant right away and there was a little bit of resentment whenever we heard someone else had gotten pregnant. It didn't seem fair.*

When I was younger, I had always figured at some point I would get married and have kids. That was just the natural order of things.

I had never imagined that it would be this difficult, or that it just might not happen at all.

Beth: It is one of the few times that I truly struggled to have any sort of faith.

On top of that, my left nipple was not looking any better.

Now, a small sore had developed in that area. It was bleeding frequently and nothing I tried - Hydrocortisone cream, Aquaphor, antibacterial cream – healed it.

Sores heal. Cuts heal.

Why was this not healing?

I finally called my OB/GYN office to make an appointment. I was running out of excuses. I knew something was wrong.

I struggled to explain the issue to the receptionist.

"It's a sore, but it's different."

I asked for the doctor who had taken such great care of me during my miscarriage hospital stay.

"She, unfortunately, is not available."

< 31 >

She scheduled me with the doctor I had seen for my annual, which I thought might be helpful because I had explained this issue to her before.

"Your appointment is September 11 at 4:00 p.m."

I hung up the phone and sat for a minute.

Everything is fine. Everything is fine.

Making that appointment, unbeknownst to me, changed the trajectory of my life.

< 32 >

5. THE MOMENT LIFE CHANGED

Beth: "It did come back malignant."

Time stopped.

Life changed.

That month leading up to this was a blur.

I remember where I was when I made THE phone call to my gynecologist's office.

> I was on my way home from school, passing the Skyline Chili and Arby's. Where we live is a US route of chain restaurants and strip malls. Our town really is "where the city meets the country." In one moment, you see rolling hills of trees with the occasional house. In another, Walmart and fast-food chains dot the view.

I had run out of excuses. Something was not right.

> I struggled to explain the issue to the receptionist. I remember saying, "It's like a sore that isn't healing. I mentioned it at my annual, but it still doesn't look any better."

> She made the appointment. The soonest she could get me in was a week later - September 11, 2018. It's funny - on a day-to-day basis, I struggle to remember little things. Chemo brain. But even now, I remember every moment of those three weeks. I remember the absolute pit in my stomach in

< 33 >

scheduling the appointment. I remember feeling really ominous... like I knew something was wrong. It wasn't nothing. At the same time, I brushed it off because I was 31. Nothing bad happens when you're 31.

The office where my appointment was with my OB/GYN was not where I usually go. I am sure it was the anxiety, but I felt like I drove forever to get there. It was red light after red light after red light. My usual office was at the hospital's doctors' building, but this was a regular medical building. It was the only place the receptionist could get me an appointment.

The OB/GYN was one I saw at my annual. I had only seen her that one time.

I laid down on the table and took my bra off - the nipple in question stuck to the inside of the bra (another reason I had called). The OB/GYN and her nurse came into the tiny room - I remember her wearing green scrubs and a smile. She asked questions about my family history with breast cancer (both my grandmothers had it twice after the age of 60) and confirmed that I was BRCA negative. My heritage is Ashkenazi Jewish descent, so there is a particular genetic mutation that seems to pop up that increases the risk of breast cancer at a young age. It is called the BRCA gene, and my former nurse practitioner had me do genetic testing three years earlier. After I received that negative reading, I thought I was off the hook.

About that...

She came in and did a breast exam on both sides, but I could tell she seemed to really consider that left breast.

< 34 >

"I don't feel anything. It looks like just a sore, but given your family history, I want to send you for a mammogram. I don't think it is anything - try some Lanolin on that sore."

By sending me for a mammogram, she probably saved my life. My oncologist said that six months could have made all of the difference. In that moment, I didn't realize that there was something growing in that breast - that sore was not just a sore.

I called the hospital from the car and scheduled the mammogram for the following Monday - September 17, 2018.

A week later, as I arrived at St. Elizabeth, Forth Thomas, I remember worrying that I was going to be late for work. That was pretty typical of my personality. Besides my marriage, my career has always been in the forefront of my self-worth. An unexpected job loss in my second year of teaching led me to Highlands High School, one of the top schools in the state of Kentucky. I put that first for such a long time.

The Women's Wellness Center at St. Elizabeth Fort Thomas is beautiful. Even though it is a hospital, it is brightly colored and welcoming. I checked in with the receptionist and waited. And waited. And waited. I went up to the receptionist and asked about the wait, explaining that I was going to be late for work. That didn't necessarily speed up the process. I remember being short with her, but I think part of that is that I was in utter disbelief that I was getting a mammogram at 31 years old.

I asked her if I could have the mammogram if I was pregnant. She said no, and I remember saying that the likelihood was pretty minimal.

< 35 >

Finally, I was walked back to a small room with lockers. I was the youngest woman sitting in that room by a long shot - probably at least 20 years. I was handed a blue cover-up to put on top... it's funny thinking about that now as it feels as though hundreds of people have now seen my chest. I waited, still concerned about the time. A friend would be covering my second period class. I remember thinking how nice of a room this was - it had soothing colors of pink and purple with neat metal vine panels.

Several people came in and out, grabbing the women ahead of me. Finally, a young woman, probably younger than me, in glasses called my name. She walked down a hallway of certificates and awards for the radiology floor. This would be a walk that I would be accustomed to over the next few months. I stepped into a room with a machine that had a plastic shelf for your breast. She explained the procedure - there would be moments I would have to hold my breath to get a good picture.

She placed my left breast on that plastic shelf and said there may be some discomfort. The white plastic piece came from above and squished my breast. I'll say it was a little uncomfortable - like someone squeezing really hard. She kept looking at the mammogram and took more pictures. I stood still and in my head, I kept telling myself that this was nothing.

But, how could a bleeding sore that wouldn't heal be nothing?

The mammogram tech stared at my pictures for what seemed like forever. I knew something was not right. I asked her innocently when I would get the results. I wanted to believe this was nothing. She said that the radiologist would take a look first, and we would go from there.

< 36 >

She walked me back to the waiting room, and again, I was checking the time. I was so afraid to be late for second period. After what seemed like an eternity, she came back and said the radiologist wanted more pictures.

My stomach dropped. Not a great sign.

My mind raced as the camera once again fell on my breast. There can't really be something wrong. I thought about the months that I waited to get this checked out. I thought about the fact that we were trying to get pregnant. After the last one of the pictures was taken, they ushered me into a conference room, one I would become quite familiar with.

The radiologist, one of the few male doctors I saw throughout this entire ordeal, came in and sat down. I've learned that when a doctor sits down, it means that this is a serious conversation.

"I looked through your scans, and I want to show you something."

He pulled out the films and pointed to what looked like to me little dandruff flakes. He called them calcifications. He said that many people have them in their breasts, but when they are clustered a certain way, it can indicate malignancy. I could feel my heart race at that moment.

"I don't think this is anything, but betting my experience with this, I think you need to get a biopsy done."

We scheduled it for the following week. I felt sick to my stomach. A biopsy... there is no way that this could actually be cancer.

I told him that we had just started trying to get pregnant again... it was our third month. He advised us to stop until this was resolved. The nausea increased.

< 37 >

A week later, I found myself in the same waiting room. Same receptionist.

I was again taken back to the same room to change. The same blue gown. I was again with people double my age.

"Beth Brubaker?"

Finally.

I was led to a large room with a metal table in the center. The table had a hole in the middle. Obviously, I knew exactly what was going there.

The technologist sat me down and asked me a bunch of questions confirming my identity. This would not be a great procedure to do for someone who did not need it. I remember she asked my birthdate, and I remember crying.

Scratch that. Sobbing.

She hugged me tightly. She was an older woman - a grandmother-like figure. I remember her saying that I was going to be fine. I said something about potentially being pregnant, and she said it would be fine - we could use two lead vests to protect that area.

The radiologist came in. She was tall and blonde... and had a soothing demeanor. She came in as I was finishing bawling my eyes out. She patted my back and began to explain the procedure. There would be pain initially, but the local anesthetic would numb it. She would collect the calcifications for testing.

"70% of the time, these are absolutely nothing."

< 38 >

The only thing I really remember after laying on the table was the initial surge of pain from medication used to numb my breast. I screamed, and the nurse in the room held my hand and promised that it would be over soon.

And it was.

I scheduled my follow up appointment for that Wednesday - September 26, 2018. I called Jason afterwards and asked him to take off. I told him that there was a 70% chance it was nothing. My heart screamed as I said those words. Fear consumed me. I shook in the car after that appointment. I do not have the greatest "gut feelings." Many of them are driven by my anxious personality.

However, in true clarity, I knew that something was not right.

In the back of my mind, I wondered if I was pregnant. I even said to Jason that this would be the month it would happen with everything else going on. Again, we had a brief window that month before we were told to stop trying, which in and of itself was devastating.

Possible but improbable.

Wednesday came.

I drove to the hospital and I met Jason in the lobby. Every fiber of my being knew that this was not nothing. Call it intuition, call it whatever you want.

I knew something was wrong.

Jason: *Truthfully, I wasn't the least bit worried. I was more focused on the upcoming weekend, during which we'd be headed to Lexington for my nephew's birthday party. I was also slightly annoyed at having to leave work*

< 39 >

early to come to this appointment. The thought that the next hour might change the rest of our lives wasn't even a blip on my mind's radar.

We checked in and then were led to a small consulting room, where a few minutes later the doctor came in.

When I saw her serious facial expression, I felt a knot in my stomach. This was supposed to be a formality, a "turns out it's nothing, just take this medicine for the next week and it should clear up" type of situation. Or so I thought.

Beth: We went up to the waiting room, and immediately, we were taken to a conference room. A nurse came in and told us that the doctor would be in a moment. What I have found is that a nurse can give you good test results. But when the doctor comes in, it usually means it is bad news.

I almost jumped when the radiologist came in. Her face looked serious, and she had a packet of papers in her hand. She faced Jason and me and said the words.

"I am so sorry, but it did come back malignant."

Time stopped.

I must have been holding my breath because I audibly gasped.

She explained that the biopsy found DCIS, which stands for Ductal Carcinoma in Situ. It is breast cancer that is essentially stuck in a duct. It is classified as Stage 0, meaning it has not spread beyond the place it started. Basically, it is the best type of breast cancer you can get. The standard treatment is surgery - a lumpectomy and then radiation. Immediately, my mind raced to pregnancy.

< 40 >

"What if I am pregnant? There is a chance I could be pregnant."

Both the doctor and nurse nodded intently and their demeanor changed to a much softer one.

"First, congratulations. Second, we can work around this."

The doctor shook our hands. We asked for a few minutes alone. I remember falling into Jason's arms and crying. I remember the words, "What are we going to do?" coming out of my mouth. We had been married a little over one year. I was 31 years old.

Jason: *Cancer.*

I couldn't believe it.

The doctor went on to explain the specifics, the plan of attack, and our options. But I don't remember most of what was said after that initial sentence. A few minutes ago, I was worried about some work project; now my wife has cancer? Is this really happening?

Beth was 31 years old. You don't get breast cancer at 31. This wasn't supposed to happen. We had been married less than two years at this point, and for the second time in five months, we were leaving a hospital with devastating news. Had we done something wrong? Did we deserve this?

Beth: The nurse came back in with a bag of information for me to look at it. She gave us the option of two surgeons that my OB/GYN had recommended. She made a comment that the female doctor had an incredible bedside manner and was based in Fort Thomas. I was sold. We scheduled two appointments — one for an MRI on Monday and then another with the breast surgeon on Wednesday.

< 41 >

Jason and I walked out stunned.

We had driven separately that day. I remember not saying a word until we reached our cars.

"What are we going to do?"

Jason said to just wait to tell anyone until we got home. It was the longest 20 minutes of my life. I remember coming home and going straight to our front porch. We started making phone calls and sending texts - a select few people knew I was going to get biopsy results. I remember thinking that I would at least be able to hide this. I wouldn't lose my hair - I wouldn't even need to tell my students. Life could stay normal.

I didn't sleep much that night. I just kept thinking about the cells multiplying in my breast. I could visualize them bursting through the milk duct and killing me. According to the informational book the hospital gave me, it explained that breast cancer is slow growing. It is actually not a "medical emergency." It can grow for 10 years before it is even noticed. However, that didn't ease my mind.

Jason: *The next couple of days went by in a blur. We steadied ourselves and prepared for what sounded like a long fight ahead, but we still were in shock. That's just not news you can process in a couple days.*

< 42 >

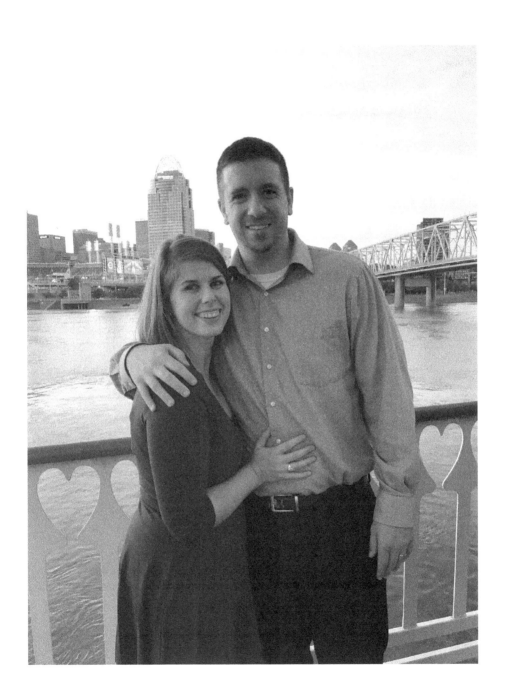

< 43 >

Beth: I went through the next two days numb. Jason and I had plans for Friday - a boat cruise on the Ohio River for his birthday. Something to look forward to. We also had our nephew's 3rd birthday on Saturday. On Friday, the surgeon's office called to remind me about my MRI.

In passing, the receptionist said, "I hear you might be pregnant. You need to take a pregnancy test before Monday... we can't do it if you are pregnant."

Pregnant... possible but improbable.

We went through our weekend with some normalcy. The boat cruise was a blast. We enjoyed a few different bourbons and saw a gorgeous sunset. Harrison's birthday was absolutely wonderful. That kid definitely knows how to brighten the day. On the way home from Lexington, I bought a few pregnancy tests from the dollar store.

On Sunday, I took one.

It didn't take more than 30 seconds to see it.

Blue plus.

Pregnant. Again.

I stared at it for what seemed like three hours.

Pregnant.

I have breast cancer.

I am pregnant.

Holy s**t.

< 44 >

I walked downstairs with the test in my hand. Jason was doing something in the kitchen - I don't remember what. My hand was shaking.

Jason: *That Sunday, Beth walked into our kitchen. I was making a sandwich; the Bengals game played on the TV in our living room.*

She had tears streaming down her face.

I then noticed the pregnancy test in her hand.

Beth: "I told you it would happen this month."

Jason: *Wait....what???*

I may have thought this, or I may have said it out loud. At that moment, nothing seemed real. My world shrunk, in that instant, to the tiny space where we stood. You could have driven a tank through our living room right then and I may not have noticed.

I likely babbled out some incoherent words that matched the thoughts racing through my brain; I don't recall. What I do remember is that we spent the next few minutes racing back and forth between tears and laughter as we tried to make sense of this.

Are we sure the test is right?

Should we be happy?

Can you be pregnant and still get cancer treatment?

Do we tell people?

Beth: Jason took the test and looked at me. I fell straight to the floor and put my back against our kitchen island. I sobbed. In the span of four days, I

< 45 >

found out that I had cancer, and that we could be bringing home a baby....
after losing one.

Two of the most extreme emotions you could feel. Jason pulled me up
and just hugged me. I don't remember what he said. He always knows the
right thing to say in the moment.

Jason: *I'd love to say that I had some inspirational words of wisdom,
delivered in a reassuring tone, which calmed us both down and readied us
for the weeks ahead. I'd also love to tell you some other lies that make me
sound more sophisticated than I really am.*

*Instead, we spent the rest of that afternoon stunned, coming up with
millions of questions and almost no answers. I didn't know the odds of being
diagnosed with cancer and finding out you're pregnant in the same week,
but I figured they had to be astronomical. We were still trying to get our
arms around the word "cancer;" now we had to plan for a baby??*

*It seemed too crazy to be true. Within the last four days, we had
received two sets of life-changing news; one frightening, the other
exhilarating. And now we had to figure out how to move forward and
balance both of them.*

Beth: We called our families immediately. My brother had already planned
to come see us that day because of my diagnosis. Now, more news. Initially,
Jason and I agreed we would wait until the end of the first trimester to share
that we were pregnant again.

However, the circumstances had changed. I was in the battle of my life
with an unexpected battle buddy. Our lives had forever changed.

< 46 >

6. BALANCING ACT

Beth: October was different. In September, I had been a teacher and wife trying to start a family with my husband.

Now in October, I was a cancer patient and a mother just praying that this baby would stick. That week, I sat in the room that we prayed would be the nursery, singing a song called "Sticky Baby."

"Sticky, Sticky baby. Mama's sticky."

Yes - very weird. Jason hated it, but for me, it was the only control I had. Our lives had changed dramatically twice in a span of four days.

One in eight women will be diagnosed with breast cancer in their lifetime, but the odds of being diagnosed while pregnant is approximately 1 in 3,000. In less than a week, I had become part of two statistical groups that no one wants to join.

That Monday, I had to call the Women's Wellness Center to cancel my MRI and tell the surgeon's office that I actually was pregnant. I also had to tell my principal, whom I had just told I had cancer, that I was also pregnant.

He probably got more than he signed up for that morning. He just kept telling me "it will be fine" and "we've got this." This was only my third conversation with him. Now, my principal knew my life story... and had watched me bawl my eyes out. There was such comfort in talking to him.

< 47 >

The call to the Women's Wellness Center introduced me to another wonderful nurse navigator who talked me down three different times throughout the day. She gave me permission to be excited about the pregnancy. It gave me hope that termination would not be on the table (from what I had already researched, that usually is not even a conversation).

Now, all I could do was wait until the first appointment on Wednesday with the breast surgeon. I had selected this surgeon based on the location (close to home and school) and the fact that she was a female. She understood the emotional part of it that was important to me. Immediately after this appointment, we would go to the airport to fly to Florida to see Jason's parents for my fall break. This was scheduled before cancer... pregnancy.... everything. It was the perfect time to get away, but of course we now had the question of whether we could even still go.

Jason: *We were obviously in desperate need of some fun and relaxation, and our annual trip to Florida seemed to be happening at the perfect time. Just a few days of relaxing with my parents....and of course taking in a Florida football game.*

We met with the surgeon on a Wednesday afternoon. Our car was packed with suitcases, just waiting in the parking lot for us to head out later that night. While working with the surgeon was obviously vital, and getting a schedule nailed down was necessary, there was still a part of me that just wanted to "get through this" and then get to the airport. We really needed a vacation and it seemed so tantalizingly close...yet here we were, in another doctor's office, with the Florida sunshine on hold for a little while longer.

< 48 >

Beth: From the moment I entered the breast center on the campus of the hospital, I knew I chose the right place to start this journey. I had spoken to many people about second opinions, but there was a feeling I got from walking in that area. It was the other side of the building where I heard the words "malignant" just a week earlier.

The same nurse navigator who talked to me on the phone so many times in the previous 48 hours was our nurse for this appointment. Jason and I figured that there was already a connection with this nurse... she had been a night secretary at the firm Jason works at many years prior to becoming a nurse. She also talked about her son and daughter-in-law finally having their miracle baby later in life. As the nurse reminded us, this pregnancy was a miracle.

The breast surgeon's honest and caring disposition struck me immediately upon meeting her. She reminded me of a mother immediately. She put her hands in mine and kept telling me that "children are a blessing" and that this was a blessing. Although there were risks of surgery, it would be safe to do it.

Since breast cancer is considered "slow-growing," the surgeon offered some options in terms of the timing. I would need a lumpectomy, which would preserve my breast and allow me to breastfeed on my other side. Then, I would complete radiation after the baby was born.

According to the breast surgeon, the benefit of radiation was still there up to a year after the initial lumpectomy.

The breast surgeon also looked at my left nipple that, again, had not healed at all. I ignorantly thought there was a difference from using the

< 49 >

Lanolin that my OB/GYN recommended, but deep down, I knew that wasn't true.

"Well, I do not think it is anything, but let's biopsy just in case."

Those words."Just in case..."

Those words.

Those words, again, saved my life.

> We tentatively scheduled the lumpectomy on October 19, 2018 at 6:00 am. That date, however, was tentative - pending input from my OB/GYN. I would see her on October 12. It was the same OB/GYN who sent me for that mammogram.

The mammogram that caught the cancer even though nothing indicated it.

With her blessing, we were in the car and off to the airport.

> **Jason:** *All in all, I thought the meeting with the surgeon had gone well. She was very personable, yet also very matter-of-fact about what needed to happen. They were going to perform a lumpectomy (which to be honest, sounds less like an official surgical procedure and more like a name you'd make up if you didn't have any medical background whatsoever, but I digress). Following that, we'd know a little more about whether the cancer had spread and what the best treatment options would be.*
>
> *While the thought of any surgery is frightening, it seemed about as straight-forward as it could get. They always have to tell you the risks and lay out the worst-case scenarios, but in that moment, I think we both felt pretty confident. The chances that the cancer had spread were minimal,*

< 50 >

Beth would no doubt come through with flying colors, and they were confident the baby would be fine.

So when we hit the road, I think we both felt a sense of calm for the first time in a while. We weren't out of the woods, far from it, but at least we had a plan in place.

And now it was time for a relaxing weekend filled with sun and sports.

Beth: Sports is something that Jason and I have always shared. If I am being honest, if I did not love sports, we would probably have not gotten married. It is truly part of Jason's DNA. I remember when we first started dating that I would check the Florida football scores while sitting in Jason's driveway before entering his house. It would give me an idea of what his mood would be.

Jason's mom said that when I told her that, she knew I was the woman for her son.

When we got off the flight, there were huge hugs and a few tears.

Thursday was a day to relax. Jason's parents have the most wonderful lanai, and we soaked in so many minutes that day. Their patio looks onto a lake on a golf course, and it truly was refreshing to the soul.

We talked about the baby... and cancer. But mostly we relaxed.

Jason: *Florida turned out to be exactly the elixir we needed after the avalanche of stress in the previous two weeks. In fact, it was almost as if everything fell into place just right, just for us, that weekend.*

On Friday, we headed to Gainesville to walk around the campus and take in the Florida/Texas A&M volleyball game. The campus was buzzing with excitement over the game the following day with LSU – you could

< 51 >

just feel it. There is absolutely nothing like a college campus before a big football game. Nothing. Just talking about it gives me chills.

But our day was about to get a whole lot more interesting.

Beth: It was quickly dubbed "Beth's lucky weekend."

Jason: *First, there was the chance encounter with the SEC Nation broadcasting crew, which always filmed on the campus of the biggest game of the weekend.*

Beth: We ran into Laura Rutledge, Jason's sports crush, and got a photo with her near the SEC Nation bus. She also took a little time to talk with us, asking us questions like "Where are you from" and "Are you excited about the game?" (I thought Jason died and went to heaven).

Jason: *Less than 20 minutes later, we stumbled on the set of the Paul Finebaum Show, which was also broadcasting from campus ahead of the showdown with LSU.*

As a college football fanatic, watching Finebaum deliver his college football takes was a reward in and of itself; however it was about to get better.

Beth: There was a break in the broadcast, and Paul was greeting fans who gathered around the set.

A producer came up to him and said he had 90 seconds until they were back on air.

Jason: *At this point, he was only a few feet from us but it didn't look like we'd get to a chance to shake his hand.*

Beth: Then, I heard a voice.

< 52 >

"Paul, I'm a high school journalism teacher. Would you mind giving my students a quick message?"

Wait - that was MY voice.

I was asking Paul Finebaum to do a video.

He said, "Sure - let's do it!"

AND HE DID.

It was AWESOME. I was so star-struck at that point. I could not believe he had seen me... and I could not believe he said YES.

Of course, I immediately posted it on our journalism Twitter account.

Jason: *It was amazing. Off the cuff, with a smile on his face...priceless. I've always been a Finebaum fan but my admiration for him went through the roof in that moment.*

Following the encounter with Finebaum, we grabbed dinner by campus and then walked over with my parents to the gym for the volleyball game. Beth is a big volleyball fan and used to coach the middle school team, so even though we'd already had an exciting day, she was pumped to see two great college teams play up close.

As we waited patiently for the gym doors to open, yet another bizarrely wonderful moment dropped right in our laps. Across the street, directly in front of the football stadium, we saw a CBS Sports camera crew gathered. They were obviously setting up a live shot, and since we had a few minutes, Beth and I wandered over to see what was going on.

< 53 >

As we got closer, we noticed them unloading what appeared to be a crystal football. I looked closely...it was a crystal football. Holy crap – that was the national championship trophy!

Turns out, they were getting some footage of the trophy at various stadiums as part of a season-long feature they were putting together. But right now, as they waited for a reporter to arrive, they were just standing on the sidewalk with the most prized possession in the sport.

One of the camera guys looked over at us.

"You guys want a picture with it?"

I tried to play it cool.

"Uh, sure. I mean, if you guys don't mind."

"Not at all – we have time to kill right now. Get right up there next to it."

What a day. At the rate we were knocking items off my college football bucket list, I expected to be holding the Heisman Trophy before it got dark out that night.

Beth: I also caught a T-shirt at the volleyball game.

2XL.....which I joked I could fill out in a few short months!

Jason: All of this, and we still had the football game the next day.

Fittingly, Florida would go on to win a thrilling matchup in one of the best game day atmospheres I've ever been a part of, just adding to our legendary weekend. A late, game-sealing interception returned by Brad Stewart for a touchdown produced the loudest crowd roar I think I have ever

< 54 >

heard. The stadium literally felt like it was shaking. To say it was amazing would be an understatement.

I don't think we could have written a script for a better time on our vacation. It was exactly what we needed, when we needed it. We both were sad to see it come to an end, but we both felt recharged. The challenges we faced were still the same as when we left. However it felt like we took on a different perspective. We were still scared but ready to face what was waiting for us.

Or so we thought.

Beth: The following week, I had my "confirmation of pregnancy" appointment with my OB/GYN after school. This appointment was important because we would need to discuss next steps and determine if October 19 was an appropriate time to do surgery.

I arrived early for the 3:00 pm appointment.

Then... I waited for TWO HOURS.

I had not planned ahead and brought food (considering my appointment time).

I was exhausted and incredibly queasy.

When the medical assistant did my blood pressure, she made the mistake of asking me how I was feeling.

"I have been waiting two hours and I feel like I am going to throw up."

They found me saltine crackers very quickly and got me to a room.

Jason was irate on the phone when I called him.

< 55 >

"That's just ridiculous. TWO HOURS LATE? Just leave."

"I can't leave - this is to confirm that we are pregnant."

He called every fifteen minutes after to check on me. I felt terrible.

> **Jason:** *Having to wait two hours for an appointment that was scheduled was unacceptable to me.*
>
> *However, perspective is always good to have. And we would learn over the coming months that running behind schedule was going to be the least of our worries.*

> **Beth:** Finally, the OB/GYN and nurse came in.
>
> This OB/GYN was the one who sent me for the mammogram. She was the one who saved my life.
>
> She apologized profusely and began asking me a lot of questions about my appointment with the breast surgeon.

"When does she want to do surgery?"

"Are they sure it is DCIS?"

She was incredibly compassionate and shared her own shock in my diagnosis.

"Not a million years did I think we would be talking about breast cancer."

> She told me that she had dealt with a brain tumor during her own pregnancy and how scary this all truly was. I cried, and she hugged me.
>
> After some discussion, she recommended I hold off on my surgery until we see a heartbeat on October 29. The OB/GYN worried I would blame myself if the surgery caused another miscarriage.

< 56 >

With the breast surgeon's blessing, we came up with an alternate date.

November 2, 2018.

The wait was truly on.

The next two weeks passed VERY slowly. The anxiety in our house was evident.

>One positive thing was seeing my journalism class officially launch the website for our student newspaper, finally completing the massive transition from print to online.

>IT WAS A HIT. Our first week, we had 2,660 hits on our website. It was such a labor of love and result of the hard work of my students. I was so proud. But beyond pride, this also would serve as an important outlet for my stress over the course of the year.

>"Typical" pregnancy symptoms began to rear their head - something that was absent during my first one.

I had horrific nausea. The only thing that would stifle it at all was eating.

I ate snacks all day long.

I also slept from the moment I came home from school to the next morning.

Finally, October 29 arrived, and Jason came with me for the ultrasound.

>The tech started the ultrasound, searched for a moment, and then we heard it.

Thump - Thump - Thump - Thump.

Heartbeat!

170 beats per minute and perfect.

< 57 >

We cried.

Correct that - WE BAWLED.

This little nugget was sticking... and appeared to be healthy.

We exhaled for a moment.

November 2 was that Friday. Life would never be the same.

< 58 >

7. GUT PUNCH

Beth: 2018 was the first time I had ever been admitted to the hospital in my life.

For 31 years, I had the good fortune to be a relatively healthy individual whose only "regular" doctor had been the OB/GYN.

In the span of eleven months, I had been admitted to the hospital for a miscarriage, then a mammogram, biopsy, multiple ultrasounds, and now cancer surgery.

The morning of my surgery, I don't remember much except that I put on my "Fight Like Fiona" shirt from Jason's coworkers (more on this later) and prayed that I would finish the surgery as nauseated as I felt now.

Yes -I am that woman who prayed for morning sickness. It seems incredibly twisted, but I knew if I felt nauseated after surgery, it likely meant that the pregnancy made it. Our rainbow baby was in the battle of its life too.

Jason: *The morning of her surgery felt surreal. Even though we had over a month to process all of the news and begin to accept it, these were still out-of-body experiences.*

When you're in the moment, you're just doing what you have to do — listening to the doctors, following their advice and being where they say you need to be. You make it about logistics to avoid thinking too deeply... "they

< 59 >

said be at the hospital at 6, so if we want to plan for any traffic and make sure we have a place to park, we need to leave by no later than 5:30. But Beth is always running late, so I'll tell her to be ready to leave by 5:20." That sort of thing.

Whatever you have to do to cope in the moment.

But every once in a while, you step back and consciously think about what is going on.

"I'm not going to work today because I'm at the hospital with my wife, who is having surgery, because she has breast cancer."

That's tough to get your head around, no matter how many days you've known about it.

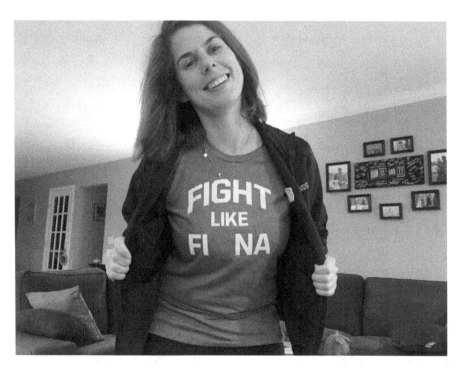

< 60 >

Beth: Jason and I arrived at the hospital at 6:00 am. The routine is the same when you go to the hospital. For a hospital, the place is incredibly welcoming. There is a person standing to the immediate left with a bright blue shirt and a smile. You walk into an atrium and go straight ahead to the registration desk. The atrium is a mix of muted tans and grey. They ask the same question first.

"Date of birth?"

"1/28/87." The number of times I've confirmed my birthdate is insane.

The woman put my bracelet on and walked us to a different set of elevators than we normally used to go to see the surgeon. Instead, these elevators were a little older, a little more rickety, and went to the surgical floor. We went down a long hallway to a place that said "Same Day Surgery."

A nurse met us and brought me to a scale to be weighed. I remember thinking that I hadn't gained that much weight in my first trimester - thanks to nausea every hour of every day. Stuffing my face with food did not seem to help.

The nurse handed me a gift bag - she said that a woman from the Women's Wellness Center had left it for me. It was pink - everything with breast cancer is always pink - and packed with essentials for a hospital stay - a brush, soap, lotion, and a few other things. I was still in denial that after today, something I genuinely love about my body - my breasts - would forever be altered.

We walked down to the pre-op room where there was a bed and gown waiting. The next few hours were a revolving door of nurses and doctors

< 61 >

asking me to sign waivers, put things in my IV, check my comfort, and talk to me about the risks of surgery and anesthesia. I think I pretty much told everyone in the hospital that day that I was pregnant. That was one thing I could control.

We waited several hours. Jason tried to take my mind off everything - we watched a movie, played a puzzle online, but mostly, we just sat - not really knowing what to say to one another.

Jason: *I remember I had a massive headache as we were waiting, and one of the nurses offered to get some Tylenol for me. She came back with Tylenol, a bottle of water and a package of peanut butter crackers, telling me I shouldn't take it on an empty stomach.*

It was a small thing — they probably have a kitchen area full of water bottles and snacks — but it was an extra gesture that she certainly didn't have to do for me. But it shows the level of caring and compassion that we've experienced with all of our doctors and nurses. If they're willing to go the extra step to make sure the husband of a patient is comfortable while waiting, you know they're going to take great care of the patient.

Beth: Eventually, the surgeon came in wearing her green scrubs. I barely recognized her. She asked if I was ready and marked my breast with a black marker - I am assuming to make sure she did the right one. I appreciated that.

About fifteen minutes later, the nurse came in and put the bed guards up. She told Jason to say his goodbyes (which to me sounded so morbid). He gave me a kiss on the cheek and told me he would see me later. I remember being wheeled down the hallway and entering the operating room.

< 62 >

Jason: *Maybe it was fatigue, maybe it was ignorance, but I wasn't overly worried when they wheeled her off. I knew she was in good hands.*

Beth: The operating room was strangely beautiful. It was bright and not as scary as one would think. The room was actually quite large. First, we made introductions - the nurse introduced me to each person in there. There were a lot of people. I remember moving onto the operating table and being told where to put my left arm. The light above me was large and sparkling. It reminded me of high school theater - the first moment of a show when the stage lights come on for the first time. I understand why they called the operating room an operating "theater." The nurse anesthetist told me that he was putting a sedative into my IV...and then...nothing.

I woke up in the room I started in. Jason was already there. I was alive. My left breast was bandaged. I was sore, but I felt okay.

The nurse helped me get dressed while Jason got the car. She wheeled me to the entrance way, and Jason took me home. I slept the rest of the weekend. That weekend felt like a waiting game. My OB/GYN scheduled an ultrasound for that Monday. Jason could go with me too for the first time. I prayed for nausea.

Jason: *I was confident everything with the baby was going to be okay. I just had a gut feeling. We had received enough bad news over the last few weeks, so maybe I was just forcing myself to believe that we weren't going to get any more today. And Beth was starting to have nausea again, which was a positive sign.*

Beth: To my relief, my nausea came back in full force on Saturday.

< 63 >

The first time I actually looked at my left breast was in the shower that Sunday. I had avoided looking at it. I was more focused on getting to Monday for my ultrasound. Then, I had to look. She had done an incredible job - just a crescent scar on my breast. Where she took the biopsy on my nipple did not look as great... which she had warned me about. I would never be able to breastfeed on that left side.... if the baby survived.

One of the first major casualties of this entire experience.

All we needed to do was see that baby's heartbeat.

We went to see our favorite ultrasound tech. She would answer my millions of questions each time she screened me.

We held our breath.

Thump. Thump. Thump.

Heartbeat.

The pregnancy made it. The baby was alive.

Jason: *There really is no feeling like hearing your baby's heartbeat. Even with everything we had been through earlier in the year with the miscarriage, and with everything we were facing now, hearing the heartbeat was a moment of pure joy.*

Beth: Tears for everyone in that room. My next appointment would be the week after Thanksgiving when I would be "officially" in the high-risk pool. I would meet my team - which included the high-risk OB nurse.

I attempted to work Tuesday, and then ended up being home on Wednesday.

< 64 >

On Thursday, I felt much better and resumed a normal schedule. Still nauseous but feeling more able to tackle my day-to-day responsibilities.

I drove home through the backroads like a typical day.

Then, my phone rang. I knew the number. St. Elizabeth.

"Hello?" I answered.

"Hi, Beth. This is the Breast Center. Do you have a minute?"

I pulled my car over. She continued.

"You have asked for us to be honest. Your biopsy results came back, and the cancer is invasive. We are waiting for more results about the type of breast cancer. We will have the results next Tuesday. I am so sorry."

The words immediately took the wind out of me.

I was going to die.

I would not see this baby grow up. I was not going to see 35.

 I was going to die.

I mumbled out "thank you" and scheduled my appointment for the following week. My next phone call was Jason. He remembers it better than I do. I was shaking.

Jason: *I got her call during a staff meeting at work. I stepped out to call her back.*

"The cancer is invasive – it's spread," she told me through tears. "I may have to do more surgery or maybe chemotherapy. I don't know what to do."

< 65 >

I hung up, quickly grabbed my things and rushed to my car. For some reason, unlike previous iterations of bad news, I didn't feel sadness or grief this time. Instead, I was angry.

Scratch that. Not merely angry. I was f**king pissed off.

Why was this happening? We had been through a lot already. We were just starting to feel a little better and catch our breath, allowing ourselves to think that the end of this adventure was almost in sight. Now we were talking more treatments and surgeries and doctor visits and hospital stays and who-knows-what-else.

It wasn't fair. How much more could we be expected to take?

Beth: I drove the rest of the way home - I don't remember how. Jason was not far behind me. That night, we just sat in the living room crying.

Jason said, "I know I tell you not to wallow - but tonight, we get to be pissed."

Jason: *I decided that maybe that night, instead of trying to put on a brave face or give a pump-up speech about how this was going to be okay, it was okay for us to just be mad. We had to let ourselves really experience it before we could move past it.*

It turned out to be pretty therapeutic. We got out some of that raw emotion so we could begin to focus on the road ahead.

Beth: My next appointment was the following week with my surgeon.

Just enough time to Google everything on the pathology report. I get emails when items are posted to MyChart.

< 66 >

....Lymphvascular Skin Involvement - Positive (basically a tumor is growing in the skin - automatic Stage III diagnosis)...

....Stage III....77% life expectancy for five years....

....HER2+....aggressive...can metastasize to brain and lung...

I sat in my classroom after school for hours staring at WebMd, Google, Healthline - the gauntlet. I just bawled.

The week felt like a million years. We just knew that I had invasive breast cancer, and it wasn't stage 0 anymore.

Jason: *I tried and tried to get her to quit looking up stuff online, but to no avail. I knew those were only giving her more ideas to fear but there was really nothing else we could do but wait.*

A few years prior to this, I had seriously injured my knee playing basketball. I remember getting X-rays and an MRI, then waiting for the doctor to come in and give me the diagnosis. As I anxiously waited in the consulting room, I thought about how some people wait in those rooms for doctors to give them news that is literally life and death. At that time, I remember wondering how anxious those people must feel, waiting for news that is much more serious than a potential knee operation.

Now, a few years later, I got a feel for it. Waiting to learn more about the new diagnosis was beyond nerve-wracking.

Beth: On the following Wednesday, I drove to see the surgeon while feeling absolutely sick to my stomach, and it was not just morning sickness. It was absolute fear - a feeling that I had never felt so strongly before. On the way

< 67 >

to St. Elizabeth in Fort Thomas, which is only eight minutes from school, I received another phone from a familiar extension.

St. Elizabeth Healthcare.

A familiar routine. I took a long breath.

"Hello?"

A different voice than the one from the Women's Wellness Center. It was the medical oncology office, calling to schedule a consultation.

That phone call meant that surgery would not fix this.

I am sure I sounded like a complete asshole to the receptionist. However, I am sure that I am not the first one or the last one.

The woman was polite, like she had heard this before.

"Our medical oncologist needs to schedule your consultation."

I guess this means chemotherapy.

I scheduled the appointment for that Friday in Edgewood - not far from school. I continued my drive to meet Jason at the breast surgeon's office, but I was so distracted. Can people even have chemotherapy while they are pregnant? (Ironically, I have been asked this question hundreds of times since).

Jason met me at the familiar atrium, and I told him that I now had an appointment with a medical oncologist for Friday. Unfortunately, he could not go with me because of work. Judi, my big sister, offered to go and be a second set of ears.

< 68 >

I declined. Too proud. I could do this on my own.

You can tell that the surgeon was a mother. I was visibly upset when I got there. My future was flashing in front of my eyes. I would die young and bald. I would not see my child go to kindergarten.

She explained her reaction to the biopsy results.

"I was shocked to see a HER2+ cancer."

You know it's a pretty crazy situation when the surgical oncologist is shocked.

We talked about what the possible treatment options would be - definitely a mastectomy and lymph node biopsy. Likely chemotherapy, which according to the surgeon, could be done during pregnancy. I could not hold back my tears.

More surgery and now chemotherapy.

She gave me a hug, and we talked about scheduling my mastectomy. I wanted to wait until the second trimester, which she was totally okay with. Then, the lymph node biopsy would tell if the cancer had spread even more.

Jason: *More surgery. Probably chemotherapy. Maybe radiation after that. We didn't get all the answers that day. But we got enough to get our heads spinning.*

Instead of maybe being close to the end of this journey, it sounded like we were just getting started.

Beth: Now, it was time to meet the next important person on this journey – the medical oncologist.

< 69 >

St. Elizabeth's Cancer Care in Edgewood was under construction to open a new building the next year. Because of the construction, the medical oncology office basically reflected the mood of the person having to sit in that waiting room.

A lot of tans and muted colors.

Bland, drab, and depressing.

I was the youngest person in the waiting room by at least 20 years. When I walked in, everyone stared.

I am not making it up - actually stared.

Young.

Pregnant.

Automatic pity party.

"Beth Brubaker?"

This was my introduction to the nurse navigator in Cancer Care. She quickly became a lifeline in the beginning of my medical oncology journey.

She walked me back to a small room. I lived in a nervous state of energy since being diagnosed, but at this moment, I felt like I was going to hurl (and not from the morning sickness).

I sat at a chair near the examining table. Again, the room's appearance reflected the mood. I pulled my laptop out to distract myself. I remember waiting a while - or maybe it just felt like that.

And a knock.

< 70 >

When I think of oncology, I think of old, crusty men who have been spending too much time looking at scientific journals. However, that's not who walked in.

A tall, long haired, young woman came in and shook my hand. Asking if I was ready, we then dove right into the plan she had for me.

I pulled out my notebook and pen to write the information down. Looking back, my scribbles made little sense, but it was a comfort to feel like I was doing something. She pulled out my pathology report. She talked through the fact that I was HER2+, and that years ago, HER2+ cancers were difficult to treat.

"Now, it is one of the most treatable types of breast cancer we have."

Cue audible breath.

She said that we now have a decision to make. Do we do chemotherapy now or wait until after the baby is born?

I think I asked the question multiple times - "Can you have chemotherapy while pregnant?" I think I also asked if the baby would live through it.

I'll tell you – she was pretty amazing at her job. She made me feel like the only patient of her day. I have thought about how hard it must be to tell someone that life will change forever.

She did an exam and said that I would see her again in a month following my mastectomy. I walked out with the nurse and scheduled the next appointment.

< 71 >

Then I walked to my car and bawled my eyes out.

This was the introduction to a huge part of my breast cancer journey. This was an appointment that, first, was an absolute blur and second, I had no business going alone. The oncologist even mentioned how impressed she was of how I handled everything. I told her that honestly, going alone was stupid, and I was absolutely wrecked.

Up to this point, only a few select people outside of family knew what was going on. Jason and I had kept it quiet except to close co-workers and friends. My intention was to keep it that way - quietly finish my surgery and radiation treatment and go on living my life.

I knew after that appointment that everyone was going to know. How could I hide my bald head at work? How could I go on making up excuses for missing school? I decided to wait to make a decision until after we had a plan in place.

So... again, more waiting.

The upcoming surgeries and inevitable chemotherapy were like black clouds hanging over our heads. It was pretty terrible - there is no sugarcoating that. Looking back, I do not remember a ton about pregnancy. This overshadowed it.

However, I do remember the day that I met a guardian angel, disguised as a nurse. It was the first appointment outside of my first trimester. Jason and I had foregone genetic testing for the baby for a variety of reasons. So the Tuesday after Thanksgiving was my first real baby appointment.

This particular appointment was so exciting because I would be able to hear the baby's heartbeat on the Doppler as opposed to an ultrasound.

< 72 >

I can't remember the OB whom I saw that day, but I remember the nurse just comforting me and telling me all would be okay. She always had a smile on her face, and always began and ended my appointments with a hug.

Then, we listened to the heartbeat. It took a few seconds, but there it was.

Thump-Thump-Thump-Thump. Fast and steady.

She said that it would get easier to find and louder to hear as the baby grew. We scheduled an appointment for the week after surgery once I met with the surgeon and the oncologist and knew more about what was going on.

However, she then did tell us to come in the Monday before my surgery to hear the heartbeat for peace of mind. Plus, Jason had not heard the heartbeat on the Doppler. We ended the appointment with a hug.

Two weeks until I would lose another part of me to cancer.

< 73 >

< 74 >

8. FINALIZING THE PLAN

Beth: The halls of the hospital had become an all too familiar place. There was a remarkable sense of efficiency - almost to the point of being mechanical. Everywhere you went, people were always moving. Sometimes moving slowly, sometimes rushing by.

Even at 6:00 a.m.

Here we were again, five weeks after major surgery. We were here again for another one. This one felt so different - so final. Today would be the day that I would forever lose a part that makes me, me. A part that makes me feel beautiful. Sexy. Hot. I absolutely loved my boobs - the way they filled out the perfect shirt. The way they gave me curves. In that same moment, I would lose the part of my body that had become an invader - a killer.

Before we left the house, Jason snapped one more picture of me in my "Fight Like Fiona" shirt. A person could barely tell I was pregnant, but a person could clearly see my chest - scarred from my first surgery, but still mine. By the end of the day, it would be gone forever.

Jason: *Watching someone you love prepare for major surgery is always scary. It's a powerless feeling, knowing there's nothing you can really do except hope the doctors do what they need to do and don't make any mistakes.*

< 75 >

And in this case, I was not only worried about Beth, but also about the baby. Heading to the hospital, I knew the next few hours could be pivotal in our lives. I just didn't know which way things might go.

Beth: Same routine - go to the registration desk. Recite my birthdate for the umpteenth time. Sign the consent to treat (like there is an option) and then sign to bill my insurance (they pretty much hate me at this point).

Then, we wait. People walk by. People rush by. You make up stories in your head about their lives... just to get your mind off what is about to happen.

"Beth Brubaker?"

We walked a similar path as five weeks ago - same elevator... same pre-op area. I got into a gown and slippers. The only benefit and consolation prize is the warm blanket.

The only difference was now there was a Doppler in our room to check baby's heartbeat. The nurse came in to do my IV - after this surgery, I wouldn't need to get an IV in my hand again. My port would take care of any blood draws or infusions. Then, the nurse attempted to find baby's heartbeat on the Doppler. She mentioned it had been a while since she had done it.

She searched.

And searched.

Nothing.

That was the most stressful three minutes of the morning. I forgot about the mastectomy. I forgot about how afraid I was. I knew it was probably

< 76 >

fine - we had just heard baby's heartbeat on Monday. However, my maternal instincts were going nuts.

After what seemed like an eternity, another nurse came in and took the Doppler.

Thump. Thump. Thump. Thump.

Baby was just fine.

Everything seemed to fly much faster than it did for my first surgery. The surgeon came in soon after and asked how we were doing.

"As well as to be expected."

She nodded. This is probably a scene she had seen time and time again. I can't imagine as a breast surgeon how hard this is. Although you are healing people, you are also taking something away.

She did the same routine - put an "x" on the left breast. Before she left, I told her something that I felt was important in that moment.

"You were the best decision I made thus far. Thank you."

Even today, that still holds true. Choosing her as my surgeon was the single smartest thing I have done in my breast cancer journey. So many decisions following that - referrals to doctors and choices in my care stemmed back to her.

Then soon after, the nurse anesthetist came in. I reminded him I was pregnant, and he said he was aware. He went through all of the risks. This wasn't just going to be sedation but actual general anesthesia. I mean - what option did I really have?

< 77 >

Only 10 minutes later, the nurse came in to take me to surgery. Similar scene - Jason told me he would see me later. His parents would be there when I woke up - they were coming to help us for the next two weeks.

Jason: *It's not exactly how anyone plans on spending December...sitting in a hospital waiting room, half-paying attention to a TV show streaming on my phone, glancing at the clock every three minutes, and wondering how things are going in surgery.*

Is Beth okay?

Is the baby okay?

They said it would probably take a couple hours...does that mean if it goes longer than two, something went wrong?

Surely they have to be getting close to being done by now, right?

Beth: Back into the operating room under the bright lights.

When I woke up, a nurse was right next to me checking my vital signs. I was in a room with patients separated by curtains. I still had the oxygen cannula in my nostrils. My brain was trying to catch up.

"Can you call my husband and tell him I am awake?"

Suddenly, I realized I was in horrible pain. The right side of my body felt like it was on fire - burning and seething. Ironically, I found that was not even the mastectomy side. It was from my port.

The nurse asked how I was feeling, and I told her that I hurt everywhere. She gave me some pain medication through my IV, and it helped

< 78 >

tremendously. Within a few minutes, a nurse came to check the baby's heartbeat.

Sure enough - it was there. Strong and steady.

Then, the radiology technician came and checked the port they had had put in place. They use a portable chest X-Ray, which I was stunned to learn was even a thing.

Then, I laid in recovery for several hours. Jason came in and sat with me... and then his parents joined us. Honestly, it was all a blur. I remember having to use the bathroom and peeing blue. Apparently, that was for the radioactive dye the surgeon used to find my lymph nodes to remove them for a biopsy.

Jason: *When I was called to meet the surgeon in a small room just off the waiting room, I don't know that I had ever felt so anxious. The surgery was finished – that much was obvious. But whatever had happened during that surgery – good or bad - was also done. There was no going back now. As I settled into a chair, I just hoped she was getting ready to deliver good news.*

"Beth is out of surgery and resting right now. Everything went fine – she did wonderfully."

I nodded and exhaled audibly. I actually hadn't even realized I was holding my breath until that moment. But the nervousness didn't disappear...there was still some other news I was waiting for.

She must have sensed that I was still anxious, because she made sure she got eye contact with me before speaking next.

"The baby is fine also. We got a heartbeat – still strong."

< 79 >

The relief that washed over me was palpable. I tried to keep a positive attitude, but I couldn't stop the worst-case scenarios from entering my mind, even if briefly.

But knowing that Beth was okay, and the baby was okay....whew. I knew recovery was going to be a long process, and then of course we had chemo and radiation to look forward to down the road. But today, right now, we were good. A big hurdle had been cleared.

Beth: There was a moment that she said I could go home that day if I wanted to. There were no rooms available, so we could wait or go home.

With the pain I was in, there was no way I could function at home... plus, I felt like garbage.

We finally made it to a room, and Jason, God love him, slept on yet another hospital cot. It was not the most comfortable night ever, and the pain came in waves. Fortunately, there were incredible CNAs and RNs to help. It reinforced my decision that there was no way I could have gone home.

A surprise visitor came to see me after surgery - the nurse navigator for my surgeon. She had been with me the day I was diagnosed and wanted to see how I was feeling, which I appreciated.

Jason: *Checking out the next morning was a great feeling. No matter how days we spent in hospitals during this journey, I never stopped being anxious when we were in one.*

I think a big part of that was just feeling helpless. There was really nothing I could do to improve the situation, to help Beth, or to make this go away. We were entirely at the mercy of others, which drives me crazy.

< 80 >

Beth: When we got home – I went straight to the downstairs recliner to sleep. I slept on and off for about 48 hours... if I wasn't sleeping, I was checking my drain output.

If you have not had major surgery before, you do not know about surgical drains.

Oh, the drains.

They are about as disgusting as they sound. A surgical drain is supposed to take fluid that comes from injury to the issue away from your body.

And you have to open them... yourself... every few hours.

The fluid is bright pink... I will never look at that color quite the same way.

Jason: I confess I did nothing with the drains. I wanted to help and be supportive, but I have a very queasy stomach about stuff like this. So I figured it was better to stay out of the way for this, rather than add to the chaos by getting sick.

I even had a hard time hearing her talk about them. I can handle a fair amount of physical pain but my stomach gets weak when you talk about medical procedures and bodily fluids.

So if there was ever a doubt about who is the strongest in our relationship, it's definitely the person who was emptying her own surgical drains.... not the guy who had to leave the room when she even started to talk about them.

Beth: Besides that, recovery went well. In a blazing moment of stupidity, I refused to take any pain medication but Tylenol. Although as the surgeon told me no less than 10 times, it was safe in pregnancy, I would not expose this baby to any more than necessary. It was painful though - your body,

< 81 >

when you lose such a heavy part. Yes, a breast is heavy if you think about it - your whole body feels off balance. Your shoulders have to readjust to this missing piece. I remember having achy shoulders and feeling hunched over.

It is not just physical pain... but emotional.

After a lumpectomy, you have a scar, but the breast is still there. After a mastectomy, there is nothing. It has been amputated. The first time you see that... you feel you are less than a woman. There is no going back.

Jason: *I knew there would be an emotional component of this surgery; in fact we talked about it frequently. My perspective had always remain unchanged....she needed to do whatever she could to get rid of the cancer to live a long life and see our baby grow up. She was not going to be less of a woman in my eyes, or in anyone's eyes. She was going to be someone who fought a difficult battle that would leave some scars, but one that she would live to talk about. That's all that mattered to me.*

But regardless of what I told her, she still struggled with the emotional pain, maybe even more so than with the physical. No matter what I tried to say, I never could find the right words to help her feel better about this.

Beth: I remember taking the outer bandage off and looking down and crying. My body was disfigured permanently. In that moment, my breasts were just mounds that existed. Their purpose did not matter anymore. My attachment to them was gone. One tried to kill me. They now just were there.

A few days later brought my follow-up with the surgeon.

She came in with the nurse and sat down. That's her thing. This woman, who is an incredible surgeon, always sits down at your level and talks to you like

< 82 >

a person. Not a patient - a person with such mutual respect. She always does her homework before she walks in.

"Well, the good news is that we think we got it all. Nothing invasive seemed to have spread outside of that initial area in the nipple. However, we ended up removing 11 lymph nodes and found micro-invasions in two of them."

Which translated to "if we had waited longer, I could be dead." In three months, we went from a nipple sore, to DCIS, to invasive cancer, to possibly spread to my lymph nodes, to an actual issue.

This was caught just in time.

My face must have been a little pale in that moment because she came closer and put her arm around me.

"You are going to be fine."

In that moment, I watched the next few months flash before my eyes - bald (a whole lot of bald), sick, throwing up, and dying. I could barely choke out the words "Thank you."

The one benefit of that appointment was... THE DRAIN CAME OUT. AND IT IS THE WEIRDEST SENSATION EVER TO HAVE IT REMOVED. (Yes - that is an all-caps sentence). From what the nurse navigator told me, people never get their drains removed the week after surgery. It usually takes more time. In my life, I have always been an overachiever... apparently in the area of drain output as well.

As always, the surgeon ended the appointment with a hug.

< 83 >

The next day, Jason and I found ourselves back at St. Elizabeth Fort Thomas to see the oncologist. Neither of us had been the Cancer Care part of the hospital, but the contrast between the Medical Oncology Building in Edgewood and this building was stark.

The reception area in Fort Thomas was beige, yes, but it had a great deal of natural light. It was much warmer. They had recently renovated it. It just had a more welcoming feeling. That may have also been that Jason was with me.

They took us back through what would become a familiar routine.

Sit in the waiting room with the bright fish tank.

Drink a cup of coffee from the reception area.

Get bloodwork from one of the medical assistants; in fact she would be the only one I found who does it painlessly.

Get weighed (and watch that baby add pregnancy pounds to Mama).

Go to a room.

Get your blood pressure taken.

Get asked if you are in pain.

Verify your medications.

Wait for the doctor.

Oh - and Cancer time. Cancer time is a real thing. In the cancer world, time moves a little bit slower. It makes sense, and I appreciate it. These people are basically giving you the worst news of your life... and with that,

< 84 >

there are bound to be a lot of questions. I know I have been on the end of needing to be consoled and asking a million questions.

This also means an appointment scheduled usually runs anywhere from 30-45 minutes behind schedule.

So... we wait.

Before this appointment, I remember telling Jason I had a feeling the oncologist was going to recommend chemotherapy while I was pregnant. I just knew it, and it made me want to throw up. As we waited for her, we both were really quiet. It was winter break, so there was no work to distract me.

Just silence. This was the scary part. This was part that you see in the movies. The throwing up, the baldness... and I was pregnant on top of this.

A knock at the door. This knock would become familiar.

"Hi Beth."

I introduced the oncologist to Jason, and she sat down by her computer. She glanced at the pathology report (you could tell she had a plan in her head already). I remember her next words very clearly.

"There was no cancer found in the breast beyond the initial area, but you had micro-invasions in two lymph nodes. We caught it. You went to your OB/GYN about this?

"Yes."

"Six months' difference... this could have been a very different conversation."

Natural next question... "So, what is next?"

< 85 >

She looked at the computer screen, and then looked at us. She rested her hands in front of her.

"Because we got this, and caught this, I don't want to let something come back if we wait. I want to start chemotherapy now."

The words tumbled out of my mouth.

"I thought that is what you would say."

Jason: *We both had kind of been expecting that news, not that it didn't still bring with it some fear and anxiety.*

We had known for a while that we were going to have to do chemo, but for a while, it seemed to be something far in the distance. We had to get through surgery and the recovery time for it, then another surgery and the recovery time for that. Chemo was like a dark cloud somewhere in our future, but we weren't quite sure when we might see it.

Now, we were seeing it. It was here.

Beth: We began talking about when. January. My first week back to school - January 10. That meant the week I got back to school, I would have to tell everyone. Everyone. -My colleagues, my students, and my parents. They would all have to know now. I had fought so hard to keep this private. The side effects of all of this would not allow me to do so. Other things came up - taking FMLA if needed, scheduling an appointment with a maternal-fetal medicine specialist to look over the chemotherapy plan, and spending time recovering from the physical aspects of surgery. It's the moment that everyone is talking around you, and you just feel numb.

< 86 >

I scheduled my next appointment - the Friday after Christmas to take part in "chemo class." This would go over the treatment plan and what to expect. Jason said more than once that this would hopefully put me at ease.

Jason: *I tried, though not successfully, to put a positive spin on it. I told Beth that though we had hoped chemo could wait a little while longer, this new plan just meant we were going to take the fight to the cancer. We weren't going to sit back and potentially let the situation decline; instead we were taking action.*

I'm not sure she entirely agreed, but I thought it was best to have an aggressive plan. The last thing we wanted was to come see the oncologist again in a few months and have her say "Oh – that's not good. We should have started this a while ago."

Beth: Christmas came and went. Jason's parents stayed with us for Christmas Eve, attending church with us and taking part in our tradition of opening some gifts that night. That tradition came from the fact that Jason and I are not patient. We did it our first Christmas together with Jason's dinky tabletop tree.

Jason's parents made that night so special, and although it was such a small gift, they gave a red Mickey and pink Minnie rattle. Jason and I had been very hesitant to tell people we were pregnant. We bought very little for the baby because we were scared. It had not even been a year since we had lost our son. However, in that moment, those rattles - it was one of the first times I felt excited and at ease that we would have a baby join our family.

Jason: *The rattles and stuffed bear my parents bought for our baby were awesome, even though they initially made me nervous. There was still some*

< 87 >

fear over what was going to happen over the next few months. Between worrying about Beth and trying to wrap my head around everything going on, I have to admit that I still didn't quite feel like I was preparing to be a parent yet.

But having my parents around to help was amazing. Beth was in a great deal of physical pain, and we were both emotionally and mentally exhausted from the prior months, causing basic tasks around the house to be neglected. Finding the time or energy to run the dishwasher or fold laundry seemed almost impossible some days.

It also reinforced just how lucky we were to have that support, to have people who were willing and able to rearrange their lives to help us out. It was never lost on us that many people don't have this option.

Beth: Christmas morning, we spent it in Lexington for the last time. Stacie, Davis, and our nephews had already purchased a home in South Carolina, and their home in Lexington was going to be sold. I know for Jason that it was especially hard. It was the last place in Lexington that Jason considered home. Now, that would be gone too.

Jason: I didn't really spend a lot of time dwelling on the fact that this would be my last Christmas in Lexington. Even though I grew up there and I absolutely love the city, I had fewer and fewer ties to it with each passing year. Many of my friends moved away and the city was growing so quickly that I barely recognized parts of it when we came to town. Perhaps that's just part of growing up — accepting change and knowing the past is exactly that.

Besides, with everything else going on in our lives, nostalgia just wasn't something I had the energy for. I just wanted us to be able to enjoy the day.

< 88 >

Beth: The day was just as it should have been - full of laughter and joy. We joined the boys in dropping parachuted plastic army men over their living room balcony, ate a lot of food, and savored some of the happiest moments we had experienced in months. However, there was such a different feeling in the air. The elephant in the room, so to speak. We knew what was coming. But even just for a day, it was nice to pretend to be normal.

We also did a very "normal" pregnancy thing - we announced we were pregnant on social media. We had waited well into the second trimester (16 weeks) because of the fear that something would happen to this baby. The fear of miscarriage never goes away.

We used our Christmas tree as a backdrop and had a colleague of mine write a sign for us - "Our greatest gift is due to be unwrapped in June 2019."

A friend and confidante in the area of pregnancy/infant loss made the perfect onesie. It was a long-sleeved white onesie with the words - "The rainbow after the storm." It had a rainbow in silver and bright colors.

At that point, few people outside of our family and inner circle knew I had been pregnant once before. Now, everyone would know. I laid the onesie in front of the sign with the Christmas tree lit up.

Then - click. Posted to Facebook and Instagram.

As we say, "Facebook Official."

Something normal - something exciting. Finally, there was a normal moment in our pregnancy. We felt incredible joy.

< 89 >

However, I opted not to tell "the other part." The biggest reason was that I did not want my colleagues or students to find out. Honestly, more than that, I just wasn't ready to admit it. I struggled to even say the words "I have breast cancer." I wasn't ready to admit it to the world.

The joy of the holidays quickly came to a crashing halt.

Friday came - back to St. Elizabeth Fort Thomas Cancer Care. This time, we would only meet with the nurse navigator for... "chemo teaching." In this meeting, she explained, we would go over the exact treatment plan the oncologist had devised. We would schedule appointments and finalize dates. All I could think walking into that building again was sheer denial.

Jason: *I knew this would not be a fun meeting. Beyond the treatment plan, we were going to get all of the details on chemo and its side effects. It's a necessary meeting — you want to be prepared for what's coming.*

But it's also tough because it all becomes real. We knew Beth was going to lose her hair. But beyond that, we didn't really know what else to expect. We only knew that we were not likely to hear anything that made us happy.

Beth: She met us in the waiting room and walked us back to a different room than before. She sat at the computer and pulled out a blue folder. Very official looking. I remember pulling out a notebook (my safety net) and a pen. She looked at us with the kindest eyes and began going through each drug.

Adriamycin... Cytoxan...Taxol...Herceptin.

Along each name came a list of some of the most horrific side effects that you could think of.

< 90 >

Complete Hair Loss. (Tears welled in my eyes).

Nausea. (I held my breath).

Vomiting. (I bit my lip to stop myself from screaming).

Mouth Sores. (I scribbled in my notebook feverishly to hide the tears).

Loss of fingernails and toenails.

That one.

> That was the one that made me lose it. I asked her to give me a minute. To beat cancer, I would have to lose my fingernails? After that, I remember little of what she talked about - there was a lot. Most of it involved calling the doctor IMMEDIATELY if I ran any sort of fever during chemotherapy. Every fever was an emergency.

All I could focus on was my fingernails. This was not fair.

> **Jason:** *The list of side effects just seemed to get worse with each minute. It felt like the pile of bad news kept growing. But what choice did we have at this point?*

> **Beth:** At the end of the teaching portion, I had to sign a consent to treat. One thing I would have to consent to was possible death from the chemotherapy drugs. It was either possible death from cancer or possible death from the drugs used to fight cancer. There was no choice in the matter. I had to do this.

> My start date was also listed. After talking to the surgeon, the oncologist decided to wait a few weeks to give me a little more time to physically recover. My start date would now be Thursday, January 24,

< 91 >

2019. It would also give me a few weeks to get things in order at school... and by things, I mean tell everyone. Tell everyone I was sick. Tell everyone I had breast cancer. Saying it made it real.

From there, we had an opportunity to see the infusion center. In the movies, it is a lot of people sitting in a single room, bald, frail looking and hooked up to IV bags. A person in the corner may be puking. Others are talking, like in a support group. This was the part I was dreading. Being pregnant, I understood there would be a lot of staring, a lot of questions, and a lot of pity. The idea I would have to be surrounded by people each week while doing chemotherapy was absolutely terrifying.

When we walked in through the door that only opens from one side, it was not what I was expecting.

Each person had their own individual treatment suite. Three walls and a curtain. I wouldn't have to talk to anyone. It was bright - a lot of windows. This area had also been recently renovated - a lot of muted pinks and frosted glass. I felt a little bit better.

"We will see you on the 24th."

This was really going to happen.

< 92 >

9. CHEMO

Jason: *The start of Beth's chemo loomed over our holidays and the first few weeks of 2019. We didn't know exactly how it would go, but we knew it was going to be a challenge. How would she feel? How would her body react? Would there be any complications with the baby? Once again, we had a lot of questions and no real answers.*

I had no idea what to expect; in fact, before we toured the chemo suite at the hospital, I have to admit I didn't even really know how chemo was administered. I had never really given it a lot of thought – I just knew it was a grueling process and there were a multitude of potential side effects, including hair loss. That was about the extent of my knowledge.

Beth: In January, our address quickly became St. Elizabeth Healthcare. Between visits to the OB/GYN and Maternal Fetal Medicine specialist and then going from pre-chemotherapy tests and follow-up appointments with the surgeon, Jason and I basically lived there. In total, there were 10 appointments - 2-3 per week... and he was at my side for just about every single one.

Jason: *Perhaps one saving grace for us was that we knew the stopping point for this round because they wanted to give her a break before the baby was due. With so many unknowns, having at least one finish line clearly marked for us was helpful in terms of our emotional state. Drawing on that*

< 93 >

inspiration, I created a makeshift calendar for Beth that showed the dates of each of her first round of treatments, also marking the days when they said she would likely feel the worst (typically 7-9 days after each treatment).

That actually became a bit of a running joke – when she would complain that she didn't feel well, I would make it a point to check the calendar to see whether that aligned with the days they told us or whether she had to wait a couple more days to complain!

We hung the calendar on the bathroom door in our bedroom so she could see every morning how much progress she had made. Being able to mark off days with a big "X" was therapeutic in some ways – a visual representation that she was moving forward, even on days where she felt she was struggling.

Beth: It began with an echocardiogram. One of the chemotherapy drugs, Adriamycin, also known as the "red devil" for its bright coloration, can cause heart toxicity in a small number of patients. Heart toxicity is a fancy way of saying heart failure. That's the death part in the waiver you sign when agreeing to chemotherapy.

We walked into St. Elizabeth Fort Thomas and went through the same routine - name, birthdate, sign patient rights, sign right to bill insurance. The front desk worker walked us to the elevator, and she showed us which floor to get off on. I truly believe St. Elizabeth makes sure the most adorable, grandmother-like women work at the front desk to check you in. They are warm, comforting, and just pleasant to talk to on the walk to the elevator.

Jason and I waited quietly. The emotional exhaustion was very real at this point. From there, we arrived in Cardiology. I purposely wore

< 94 >

a baggy sweatshirt to avoid the stares. A slender blonde woman with glasses came out.

"Beth Brubaker?"

Jason and I both stood up and followed through the gray metal double doors. There was an audible click behind us.

We walked into a darkened room complete with a hospital gurney and machine that I immediately recognized. A few years back, it was discovered that I have an "innocent" heart murmur. It has not caused an issue, but I did have an echocardiogram done a few years back. I laid down on the gurney and got undressed from the waist up - I had JUST begun to show a little bit, and the sonographer took notice.

"Just so you know I am pregnant if that makes any difference in the test."

She smiled and said it didn't. We chatted more. I told her what I did for a living, and we discovered her son attended the high school where I taught. She was so sweet - she promised she wouldn't tell him we met. I said it was okay.

She attached the electrodes to my skin and had me lay on my side. My protruding bump was more obvious at that angle.

We finished, and she wished me good luck with everything.

The next day, we visited another hospital to meet the Maternal Fetal Medicine specialist and learn the gender of the baby. This felt like something normal - something actually fun about being pregnant. Jason and I had toyed with not finding out or not telling people once we did... but curiosity and excitement won out. I had a grand plan that I would get two

< 95 >

cupcakes from an adorable little bakery near the hospital. The baker would fill it with pink or blue... in my head, it would be adorable.

Jason: *Beth had been saying for weeks that she wasn't sure she wanted to find out the gender, that she wanted to be surprised in the delivery room. For me, it was never even a question. There was already so much I didn't know, so many questions I had, so I wanted to eliminate any uncertainties as soon as possible.*

I have a ton of respect for expectant parents who can live with that uncertainty until the baby arrives...but no way could I have handled that.

Beth: The Maternal Fetal Medicine Center is clear on the other side of the hospital. It has the most beautiful frosted windows, and for being a waiting room, it is a calming place. But as most appointments in the medical world go, they were running late... and Jason needed to make it to work.

Finally, they took us back, and the sonographer laid me down and began the anatomy scan.

It was incredible.

Every part of this tiny human was formed and perfect. Every feature resembled an actual human. That moment was beautiful. This little one was for real... really there.

The sonographer showed us every part.

Every finger.

Every toe.

Every vertebrae in the spine.

< 96 >

The grooves of the brain.

God's work.

> She told us to turn away as she looked at the gender. I squeezed my eyes shut. Butterflies filled my stomach... which ended up being the baby kicking (which I didn't realize yet).

> From there, Jason and I were escorted to meet the Maternal Fetal Medicine specialist.

We waited.

And waited.

And waited.

> The room's walls had bulletin boards covered with Christmas cards and birth announcements. It was like a miracle baby hall of fame. I could not wait for OUR baby.

> **Jason:** *It was a very surreal feeling to look at all of the pictures of babies in there and realize that we were soon going to have a baby ourselves.*

> *With everything else going on, there were still times it didn't seem quite real yet. But that day, seeing the sonogram and knowing we were going to find out the gender, it felt more real than ever before.*

> **Beth:** An hour and half later, Jason had to leave for work, which meant I would need to absorb all of this information by myself. The maternal fetal medicine specialist's job was to check the oncologist's plan for chemotherapy to ensure that the baby would be healthy.

< 97 >

Finally, the MFM specialist walked in. She quickly shook my head and sat down, clicking quickly on the computer screen. Everything with her was fast... her matter-of-fact tone included. She flipped through the printed file... fast.

I also learned that with her matter-of-fact tone came a little bit of sassiness, which I appreciated so much.

"Well, this is really shitty, isn't it?"

I was not expecting that question but answered with a resounding YES.

She repeated each step of my chemotherapy journey - every drug's name, every length of time, and then the ultimate goal - delivery at 34-37 weeks.

She mentioned she would send a report to the high-risk OB nurse, and we would go from there.

Then, we were done.

Walking out of the hospital, I transformed into a typical pregnant woman. I proudly carried the ultrasound envelope, which bore a very appropriate Bible verse: "You are wonderfully and fearfully made." (Psalm 139:14)

I felt like a real mom.

With a newfound pep in my step and the feeling of holding this incredible secret, I went to the bakery. This bakery has been in business for over 50 years, and the interior reflects that. The yellow walls were lined with old-fashioned baked good cabinets with fresh donuts waiting to be plucked from them. The smell of the place was reminiscent of fresh bread. I was nearly without morning sickness, so I soaked it in.

< 98 >

I laid my purse on the counter and explained the situation. The woman was so kind and said normally they would need a few days. I must have had a look of desperation because she went to the back and came back grinning.

"Can you give us an hour?"

UM. YES.

> **Jason:** *It was very tough to focus on work that day. Knowing that life-changing news was waiting for me at home made me more anxious than usual to get the work day over with.*

> **Beth:** I ran out to do another typical pregnant lady thing... satisfy a craving. Throughout my pregnancy, the two cravings I had were sweets (which the old wives' tales say means GIRL) and Frisch's Big Boy sandwiches. I had more Big Boys during my pregnancy than I ever did prior to that... and I worked at Big Boy to put myself through college.

Fortunately, I knew that there was a Frisch's Big Boy close by.

> I sat down in the booth and quickly ordered. I savored that Big Boy with butterflies in my stomach (either baby kicks or excitement over the gender... not sure which). The time went by so slowly. All I wanted to do was pick up these cupcakes and speed time up for Jason to come home and see if my gut was right.

> After what seemed to be an eternity, I skipped out of Frisch's and drove to the bakery. The cupcakes were waiting for me. The baker had gone above and beyond. She decorated each one with white frosting with dots of blue and pink. She even had wrapped it in special pink and blue paper. I had just left an appointment where a doctor went through scary drugs that could, in

< 99 >

theory and, if administered incorrectly, harm our child. But in that moment, I didn't care. I was going to find out if we were having a son or daughter by cutting into a really cute cupcake.

Those moments of sheer joy were few and far between.

I have no idea what I did to kill four hours before Jason came home. The cupcakes sat on our kitchen island, and I just stared at them. The ultrasound envelope sat on top the cupcakes, taunting me.

Finally, the garage door opened, and Jason walked in. We had dinner, and then we both sat down with our respective cupcake. On the count of three, we agreed to cut and open them.

We both just smiled at one another.

"1... 2... 3..."

Cut. Open.

PINK.

We were having a little girl. There was no debate anymore if this was Hayden Jay or Harper Jaye.

Our nugget was Harper Jaye Brubaker.

I looked at Jason, got up and hugged him, crying. I also said, "I knew it!"

Jason: *Beth had been saying it for weeks — she just had a feeling we were having a girl. I always joked that I needed to have a boy because I had no idea how to raise a girl.*

< 100 >

But seeing that pink frosting was a pretty amazing moment. We were going to be parents to a little girl. That realization washed over me like a wave; in fact, it was probably the first time in this journey that I really felt like a parent.

No longer were we waiting for a baby. We now were waiting for Harper.

Beth: We took a picture and sent it to our families first. Everyone was so excited. We already had two amazing little boys in our family... and now a GIRL. It was a necessary light for the coming week.

This week would be my "prep week," so to speak. This would be the week I would get fitted for a wig... and that "my dirty little secret" would become public to my colleagues, my students, and their parents.

My appointment with the Women's Boutique at St. Elizabeth was on Tuesday. I would get to see the woman everyone called "Chick." I knew her from the breast cancer organization she started in Northern Kentucky, "Chicks 'n Chucks."

I sat down at the desk at the Women's Boutique. The boutique itself reminded me of my grandmother's sitting room. It was covered in knick-knacks. It had a pink tint to it, and overall, it was just warm. Honestly, it may have been because of Chick and her partner-in-crime in the boutique, Bubbles. She sat behind the desk and began going through the "business" part of all of this - insurance, etc. I would be fitted for a prosthesis for my missing breast and then a wig for hair loss during chemotherapy.

< 101 >

First, the prosthesis - the fake boob. I had been wearing a "knitted knocker" as they are called, but the breast surgeon said that not having a natural weight could cause back issues. Chick fitted me and ordered it.

Then the wig. A true acknowledgment of what was happening.

School has always been a safe haven for me. More like my sanctuary. Life made sense at school. Every day was the same routine - a perfect scenario. You pour yourself into a common good - teaching young minds to hopefully make them better people. It is truly a calling. There is a sense of perfection. My role as a teacher felt sacred. My personal life, although there were moments of intermingling, toed the line of my teaching persona.

That moment was about to change.

Jason: *I knew telling everyone at school was a huge step for her. She didn't want to be treated differently, looked at differently, pitied...any of that. But once you deliver news like this, it's inevitable that will happen.*

I just tried to prepare her for that, while also emphasizing the positives. Namely, that she was getting ready to gain a ton more support in her battle. She is well-liked and respected at the school, and knowing some of her colleagues, I knew they would step right up to walk beside her in this. But I also knew that it was still scary to make public news that was so personal for us.

Beth: I met with my principal multiple times to read over the email I would send to my colleagues. I had my department chair, who happens to be one of my closest friends, read it as well. My plan was to send it on Wednesday as I was leaving for the day. My colleagues already knew I was pregnant

< 102 >

from our December faculty meeting, but they did not know the rest of the "news."

Wednesday came more quickly than I had hoped. The bell rang at 2:45 pm. I opened the drafts of my email and just stared at the words in front of me. My eyes scanned them again.

Dear School Family,

This is an incredibly difficult email for me to write. However, I feel considering my next steps that this was an appropriate time to share with all of you a health issue I have dealt with this school year.

This past September, I found out that I had an early-stage form of non-invasive breast cancer. They found it early thanks to my wonderful doctor. The initial course of treatment was going to be surgery and radiation. We found out the news of my pregnancy four days after this – talk about timing.

In November, I went in for surgery, and the surgeon opted to do a biopsy of another spot that I had been concerned about. She didn't think it was anything but wanted to make sure. In that spot, they found a small spot (very small - 6 mm) of invasive breast cancer – again, caught VERY early. However, this meant more surgery, including checking my lymph nodes to see if it had spread. This also meant I would need chemotherapy of some sort – a change in the initial plan.

I had another surgery in December (which is why I missed the last week of school before winter break). The pathology report, thankfully, showed very little invasive cancer had spread. However, in two lymph nodes (out of 11 removed), there was a "micro-invasion" of invasive

< 103 >

cancer - again, caught early and removed. It appears that between the two surgeries, all of the cancer has been removed.

That being said, my oncologist wanted to wait until after the December surgery to see about next steps for chemotherapy and timing. Because right now the cancer is, in her words, "curable," she does not want to wait to start chemotherapy until after the baby is born. I will begin chemotherapy on Thursday, January 24. It will be every three weeks for four sessions, stopping eight weeks prior to my scheduled delivery. I will then do more treatment following that. Jason and I are still amazed that yes - you can be pregnant and have chemotherapy with little risk to the baby. I'm in great hands - my oncologist, surgeon, OB, high-risk OB nurse, and a maternal fetal medicine specialist from Good Samaritan Hospital are making sure our baby is healthy and developing normally. She is - measuring perfectly at 18 weeks!

I felt compelled to now share this information with you, my Highlands family, because obviously, with chemotherapy, there are side effects that will be noticeable, including losing my hair. We have worked out a plan that I will be able to continue teaching during treatment - maintaining that ever important normalcy in my life, which is needed for a successful recovery.

Again, I apologize for not sharing this information sooner - to be honest, it's been an incredibly difficult time for Jason, myself, and our families. Plus, school has been one of the few places that I felt normal during a time when nothing in our lives has felt that way. I also wanted to make sure that my students did not find out before I was ready to tell them. All they know is that I have needed surgery. I will do that in

< 104 >

the next few days, as well as telling my students' parents. I do please ask that you allow me the opportunity to share this information with my parents and students on my own time.

Your prayers are appreciated, and I will keep everyone updated as I move forward through treatments this spring. We caught this early, and Jason and I have said from the beginning that this is a bump in the road for our family. We are looking forward to this time next year having a healthy baby girl and me being cancer free.

Thank you so much. I truly appreciate all of the support and help in advance.

Beth

Deep breath in. Release.

Thump-thump-thump. My heart pounded in my chest.

I packed my school bag up with the exception of my laptop. I stared for a few more moments. Tears dripped down my face.

Just a few more moments of normalcy.

Click. Swoosh. Sent.

I threw my laptop in my bag and ran out of school, avoiding eye contact with anyone. These were the days I was grateful for a long car ride home on the backroads of Kentucky. I could sob the entire ride and just decompress.

That's exactly what I did.

I lost a piece of innocence in that moment. School was no longer a safe haven. There was no normal place in our lives anymore.

< 105 >

I did not check my email that evening. Though I knew people would send well-wishes, and though they were appreciated, I was not in an emotional place to read them.

Upon my arrival to school the next day, I stayed in my room most of the day... but my door became a revolving one with people offering hugs and support. At one point, I had to ask one of my colleagues to leave because I did not want to cry in front of my students. I also had spent most of the off minutes of that day drafting an email to my students' parents. I wanted them to know first. Every student carries emotional baggage, and even though we may not be able to see it outwardly, it is there. I did not know if cancer had touched some of their parents or grandparents, and this news could be devastating for a student like that.

The email was similar to what I sent my colleagues, only with more benign information. The biggest thing that I wanted to know is if there were students dealing with cancer in their families. I wanted to be able to look out for them.

I sent that email early in the day, and within minutes, I had responses. Stories of some devastating diagnoses within families. Prayers and requests of what parents could do.

My heart was in a million pieces after those two days.

And Friday was still to come.

Friday. Friday, my students would know.

All of the generalizations about my surgeries would make sense.

All of my absences would be clarified.

< 106 >

That night, I told Jason that I would allow them to ask any questions they wanted. I wanted them to feel like I would be honest with them and not sugarcoat anything.

I slept very little that night.

Jason: *I think she was more nervous to tell her students than she was before either of her surgeries. Being a teacher is everything to her, and though she prides herself on being able to relate to her students, I knew she was worried about being that vulnerable in front of them.*

I talked to her about the fact that her story was not going to be one of sadness, but one of inspiration. That her students were going to see her courage and toughness, and remember that for years to come in their own lives. That her actions now could shape their attitudes long into the future.

Beth: I took the long way to school that day. An extra turn here and a backroad there. It was pitch black outside and quiet. A calm before a storm.

Usually, mornings in the car were full of podcasts and music. This morning, nothing felt appropriate.

In my classroom, you can rarely find me sitting. I am constantly moving. An office job would be purgatory. Even at 18 weeks pregnant, my butt barely touched a chair. However, I have this broken stool from one of my former colleagues. I have never fixed it....out of forgetfulness or laziness.

But my students know that when I sit in that chair, the door shuts, and it means a real conversation.

With each class, I took a deep breath and soaked in a moment. Some of these students I knew since they were sixth graders from coaching, from

< 107 >

having their siblings, from relationships with their parents. Even if they thought I was a challenging teacher, had unreasonable expectations, was no nonsense, they were all still kids. For some of them, they had never been around a person who was sick before. Even if I was not their favorite teacher and they just tolerated me, this was going to be hard for them to cope with.

"Some of you, I know, have spoken with your parents...."

I had a scripted beginning, one that I had worked on in my head since the day I was diagnosed, prepared if this moment ever came.

"I am sure some of them have spoken to you about what I am going to share."

This was the moment.

"As you know, I had a few surgeries this fall, and the reason for those surgeries is that they have diagnosed me with breast cancer."

Pause. My internal dialogue screamed "HOLD IT TOGETHER."

I explained my treatment plan to them. Some of them had tears in their eyes. Some just wore shocked looks.

Each time, I opened it for questions. I really encouraged them to do so. A few asked if I was scared. I answered honestly - YES. One student asked about breastfeeding (never in a million years did I expect that to come up), and I was honest that I could not.

There were two moments that were particularly hard that day.

First involved a student whom I had as a sixth-grade volleyball player. She was now a sophomore in my English class. Prior to leaving my class that

< 108 >

day, she just looked at me and gave me a hug. She cried, and I fought back tears. I knew that one would be hard.

The next moment was seeing my sixth period class. This was my only junior class of the day. There is something special about teaching juniors. They are actual adults. This class comprised 18 of the most special young people whom I have ever had the pleasure to teach. As a teacher, you want to build that family atmosphere in a classroom. With this group, I truly had that. Everyone looked out for each other.

As I explained the situation, their faces were like stone. I will never forget. Finally, one of them spoke up.

"Mrs. Brubaker, we have your back. We are here for you."

The tears I fought all day finally came through. Before the day started, my colleague said that I was giving them a lesson on life... what it is like to push through even when things are terrible. That moment really showed me that.

That night, Jason and I went to see a movie, and while he drove, I just sobbed. Everyone knew. Life had changed.

However, in those tears, came relief. Relief that I didn't have to lie anymore. Relief that I could actually feel some emotions around others.

In the days following, the anticipation towards January 24 began to build... like this volcano simmering until it erupted. With all of this happening, I began to feel other things in my stomach - a feeling I had never had before. Almost like butterflies. It happened more when I was laying on my side. Our black lab, Percy, would paw at my stomach gently - like he knew.

< 109 >

At my OB/GYN appointment, the doctor and high-risk OB nurse confirmed that I was likely feeling Harper kick. It was incredible. I would shake my stomach just to feel her swishing around in there. It meant that she was developing normally. She was perfect.

The weekend before I began chemotherapy, Jason booked a trip to Gatlinburg as a "babymoon" for us. We had this incredible cabin complete with a hot tub (that I couldn't use) and the most sensational view of the forest. It was picturesque and a complete contrast to the current state of our lives. We ate at some great local restaurants, played mini-golf, went to the Crime Museum, and the last night we were there, it snowed. It made the fact that no pizza place would deliver to our cabin trivial in the grand scheme of things.

It was the first trip we had taken alone since our honeymoon and likely the last by ourselves for a long time. But as wonderful as the trip was, there was a feeling of impending doom. A precipice of an unknown. Although we went through two surgeries, this felt different. This felt like the turning point.

Jason: *It was a strange trip. On the one hand, it was very relaxing, very low-key, and just what we needed at that point. But on the other hand, it felt very much like the dreaded "calm before the storm." It was never far from our minds that this might be the last weekend in a long time where things felt even somewhat close to normal.*

Beth: Thursday came quickly.

Very quickly.

My students, the day before, brought me flowers and cards.

< 110 >

I took the entire day off work because we did not know what the outcome would be. The plan was that I would return to work on Friday, and then take the weekend and just see how I felt.

I barely slept Wednesday night. At this point, I was 20 weeks pregnant and beginning to show. Sleep was difficult to come by anyway, but that night, it was non-existent.

My appointment was early. I pulled on my "Fight Like Fiona" shirt and packed my "chemo bag" full of blankets and warm socks. I tied my hair back. My hair that would soon be gone. Waiting for Jason to get ready, I sat on the couch and bawled. Like many times before, I asked out loud, "Why is this happening to me?"

Jason came in, and he snapped our usual picture with me and my shirt. I held up a 1, and my pregnant belly was evident. That "Fight Like Fiona" shirt fit just a tad more snuggly than it did in December. The tears welled in my eyes, but I still had a smile on my face. I even wore a pink zip-up sweatshirt because... everything with breast cancer is pink.

< 111 >

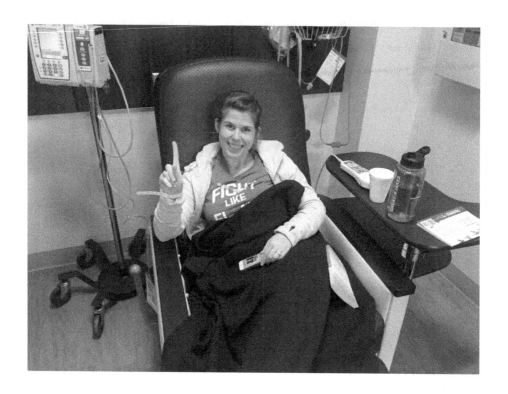

Everything from leaving the house until reaching Cancer Care was a blur. There were more tears in the car, but otherwise, it was a quiet ride. Neither of us knew what to say.

We arrived and moved into the familiar waiting room at Cancer Care. I would see the oncologist first, and then would begin my first chemotherapy treatment.

Jason and I were just quiet. Quiet while we waited, quiet before she came in.

When she did come in, she asked the obvious question of how I was doing. I mumbled some garbage of just wanting to get this over with. Inside, I was dreading every second. It was one of the most terrifying days of my life. She

< 112 >

went over the protocol of the day, and then the following week, I would see her just to see how I was doing.

My mind was racing.

We are not actually going to do this. We are not actually going to do this.

The oncologist walked us to the waiting room. I just stared at the door. The door to the infusion room. The door that does not open from the waiting room - you have to be let in. A wave of nausea came over me. This was actually going to happen.

We sat for a few minutes before one of the infusion nurses called us back.

She escorted us to a room right in the middle of the other rooms. Total in Fort Thomas, there are 10. The room is tight quarters - a brown wall in the back with all of the machines plugged in - IV, blood pressure, and a few others. They divided the rooms with frosted glass on each side - it was pretty... calming. The front was open with a curtain that could be drawn.

We waited for the infusion nurse to come in. She was in part-time, and her day happened to be Thursdays.

With every injection of my premedication, which included Zofran and steroids, I asked questions... a lot of questions. Even though I knew three pharmacists had looked at every medication I was receiving, I still asked again.

How will I feel?

What will this do?

< 113 >

When will it wear off?

The nurse calmly answered each question down to the last detail. She also warned about that ONE steroid that makes your crotch area burn like mad.

Then came waiting for the pharmacy. Chemotherapy medications cannot be mixed ahead of time because it is so expensive. They wait for your blood counts to see if you are well enough to do it. After it is mixed, it is HAND DELIVERED to a locked closet to then be administered.

The nurse brought two plastic bags over. Both were marked with a bright yellow label that read:

DANGER - CHEMOTHERAPY.

Complete with the cytotoxic hazard symbol.

Yep - the liquids in those bags were going into my body...with my baby growing in there.

She got dressed to administer the drugs - a full gown, plastic gloves, mask - everything. She also had another nurse check the drugs and patient's name to make sure everything was where it should be.

Jason: *It's more than a little disconcerting to see the nurses put on full hazmat suits just to handle a bag, the contents of which will be going into your wife's body. I wondered how on Earth it could be safe for Beth or Harper if they couldn't even touch the bag with their bare hands.*

But we had to just trust they knew what they were doing, regardless of how surreal it all seemed.

< 114 >

Beth: First, a large push syringe with a bright red liquid in it. This one was the reason I needed a port in my chest. This was the dreaded "Red Devil."

It had to pushed VERY slowly because it could eat through your skin, kill you, etc. The nurse also mentioned that this makes you pee red for about 48 hours, and that Jason and I could not share utensils, or be intimate (no sharing bodily fluids) for 48 hours too.

As she pushed, I expected to feel different. Like the world blew up.

I didn't.

Then, the nurse hung a clear bag. This was Cytoxan, another chemotherapy drug often paired with Adriamycin. It would drip for an hour.

I did some schoolwork, ate pretzels, and drank a Sprite while the fluid dripped. This became almost a ritual. They warned me to keep it light the first day because I wouldn't know how I would react. Sprite and pretzels became my snack of choice. Jason worked on something on his computer.

Then - *beep. Beep. Beep.*

I was done. I would be back for my follow-up appointment the following week. It felt so anticlimactic - I expected to be nauseous or something. Instead, I just felt tired because I had been so amped all week.

Jason drove us home, and I laid down the rest of the day.

I went to school the next day like nothing happened. I taught my classes and came home to sleep.

That was basically the theme of the weekend. I did not move out of bed for most of the weekend. I had never felt so tired in my life. The effects of

< 115 >

the chemotherapy were starting to kick in. My body was being overwhelmed with drugs that were destroying every dividing cell in my body.

The only concern I had was that I could feel Harper shaking in my stomach. We figured out, after calling my OB/GYN, that was probably from the steroids. It still was a point of anxiety.

Jason: *The first treatment was a huge hurdle for her to clear, not just physically, but also emotionally. Though we knew the effects were cumulative and would build over time with each chemo session, we at least now had a baseline. We had an idea of what it was like and how she would probably feel. Some of the uncertainty was gone, which was a welcome feeling.*

Unfortunately, one certainty was still looming like a black cloud.

< 116 >

10. HAIR LOSS

Beth: With the first chemotherapy session over, we now knew what to expect.

First day - feel fine.

Second day - jittery and debilitating fatigue.

Third day - can't move out of bed.

Fourth day - struggling to get up and go to work.

> But by a week after chemo, I felt (dare I say it) normal. I did not have any nausea after the IV medication wore off. The two anti-nausea medications just sat in their respective orange bottles. Even the nurse navigator, when I spoke with her the Monday after, seemed surprised.
>
> What also surprised everyone - us, the oncologist, and my OB/GYN - is that my white blood cell count stayed in the normal range for a pregnant person. Adriamycin and Cytoxan are known for absolutely decimating the immune system. A fever is an emergency.

My counts, however, stayed normal. God was looking out for Harper's well-being.

> Another week passed after finishing my first chemotherapy. Life went on. I looked normal. My belly continued to grow. Instead of just looking fat, I began looking like I was pregnant. On the outside, you would never know what was happening.

< 117 >

Until February 1, 2019.

I first noticed it in the shower. Strands of hair began slipping through my fingers. My dark brown hair contrasted with the bright white floor of the shower.

It was happening.

You know it is coming.

It does not make it any less traumatizing to see.

Nothing prepares you for that.

Another reminder of my body being under attack.

Jason: *She was, understandably, distraught. The most distressing aspect for her was that it would be a very visible sign of her cancer. Up to then, Beth still looked completely healthy. If you didn't know her, if you passed by her in the grocery store or saw her in the line at Starbucks, you'd never guess the battle she was waging.*

But losing her hair would be different. Now, everybody would know, or at least be able to guess. If you see someone her age with no hair, your brain almost automatically makes the connection that this person must be sick, likely some form of cancer, and they've lost their hair because of it. And that assumption then leads to sympathetic stares or hushed whispers, which might come with the best intentions, but also reinforce that something is different.

The last thing she wanted was pity or to be treated differently.

< 118 >

Normalcy was something we tried to maintain to the best of our ability, but it was quickly slipping out of our grasp.

Beth: Over four days, my hair thinned at an alarming rate. I would pull it up to hide the patches of scalp beginning to show through. Jason said he could not tell.

But I could. I was embarrassed and sad. Towards the end of that week, I finally called my hairdresser. She knew that the call was coming. We talked about it in November. This woman had been cutting my hair for seven years. She did my hair for my wedding... and now, she would shave off that same hair for my cancer treatment.

Yeah. What a contrast.

I made her promise that no one else would be there. The stares of being pregnant and going to the Cancer Center were enough. I felt shame. Shame that was happening to me. Even though we had told our friends, family, and colleagues, I still felt such an unease about what was happening. Like I was watching another person go through all of this.

Jason: *Beth decided a few months earlier to shave her head when her hair started to fall out. And though I couldn't really tell that it was thinning out yet, I also knew this was something she had her mind set on doing. There wasn't a lot we could control in our situation, but this was something she could do. She would not let cancer take her hair. If she was going to be bald, she was going to do it on her terms.*

Beth: I walked in the historic building where my hairdresser is located. The bell clanged against the door as I opened it. Peering around, my hairdresser

< 119 >

met me with a sad smile. We hugged for a brief instant, and I took off my sweatshirt.

"Are you okay?"

I smiled weakly.

"Let's do this."

As a final act of kindness towards my hair, she led me over to the sink, and laid my head down. I could hear the pump and squirt of the shampoo, and then felt her fingers along my scalp. Even though she knew what she was about to do, she still took the time to treat my hair with dignity and respect. Her fingers massaged my scalp - there is truly nothing like having someone else wash your hair.

And this would be our last appointment together for at least a few months.

We both started to cry. We made normal conversation - asking about how I was feeling and if I had felt the baby kick. She has three of the most beautiful girls; the youngest had just been born when she began cutting my hair. Small talk to escape the elephant in the room.

After washing my hair, she led me over to the chair, and as always gave a small neck massage with the most incredible smelling oil.

Then, the buzzing started.

I could feel the clippers graze against my scalp, and with each stroke, a strip of hair fell to the ground.

Buzz.

Another strip.

< 120 >

Buzz.

Another strip.

Until there was none left.

> We talked throughout, but I can't remember what was said. Honestly, we talked in order to keep ourselves from crying.

I looked in the mirror and took a breath. I held back hot tears.

Strangely, these words tumbled out of my mouth.

"I look like my brother."

As I went to grab my wallet, she stopped me.

"You are not paying for this."

> We both started to cry, and she gave me one more hug. I put on the headscarf I had brought, and went to the car. No one was outside, but in my head, I felt like people were staring at me.

My appearance now reflected my illness. There was no hiding now.

> I walked in the door with my headscarf, and Jason was sitting in the blue armchair in our living chair.

He said, "All right, let's see it."

> I took it off and just collapsed in his arms. I was sobbing. He kept telling me how badass I looked, how beautiful I looked, but in my mind, I just looked sick.

< 121 >

We took the "after" picture on the couch with me holding Scout. Scout, our dachshund, had been with me since my first year of teaching. Before Jason, he was the only man in my life. In that moment, he just rested his head on my lap... grieving with me. Dogs have such an incredible sense about that.

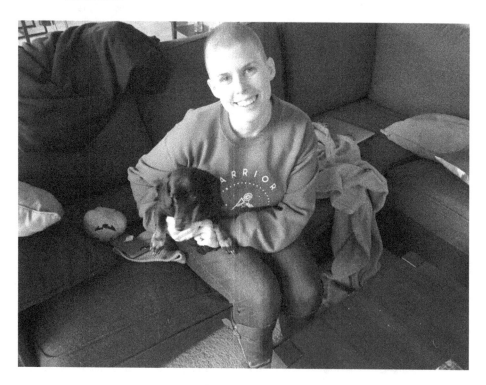

Purposely, we had made dinner reservations that night at a fantastic Italian restaurant, thanks to a birthday gift card. We were treating this like an early Valentine's Day dinner because I had chemotherapy on the actual day (great planning). I put on a black dress that showed my ever-growing bump and bought a purple scarf and earrings. Finally, it was a decision about headwear.

< 122 >

Wig or headscarf?

Something about my wig made me like I was trying to hide everything...
again, like there was this shame associated with going through cancer
treatment.

I pulled out a black, sparkly headscarf that another survivor from an
online support group had sent me. It was covered with sequins - it was fun!

I remember coming out of the bathroom, and Jason just looking at me.
He smiled and said, "You look awesome."

We went to dinner, and while we waited for our table, someone
snapped a picture of us. We truly looked like a normal couple, just with
a headscarf. The true test would be going to school on Monday with a
different appearance. I had warned the kids ahead of time that this was
coming, but my nerves were raw thinking of it.

The weekend came and went quickly.

It rained that morning.

Rain and a wig sounded like a terrible combination. I threw on a headscarf,
and I went to school. That wig ended up sitting in the box for months.

I taught a normal day. Not one thing was said to me. It was the
elephant in the room, and not one person wanted to deal with me -
myself included.

At the end of the day, as I packed my bag to leave, one of my students
came in. She looked at me and smiled.

"I just wanted to tell you how wonderful you looked today."

< 123 >

And then just left.

I made it 30 seconds before I started crying. Someone had acknowledged what had happened. It made my heart grow 50 sizes. It gave me some confidence. It gave me the acknowledgement.

Things returned to normal - kind of. As normal as they can be when you are pregnant and going through chemotherapy. Between ultrasounds and doctors' appointments, I was missing classes left and right, but I was grateful that I could continue to teach.

The week of my second chemotherapy treatment came at a roaring pace, and again, it was scheduled for Valentine's Day. My doctor's appointment would be with the nurse practitioner at the Cancer Center. I told Jason jokingly that even the oncologist had made better plans for that day. I would leave school at 11:00 a.m. to go have treatment.

I walked to my room and noticed a chain of paper hearts strung around my door. They were differing colors and sizes, but they each looked like a small valentine.

And then from the moment my keys clicked to unlock everything, the revolving door began.

Envelopes of valentines. Flowers. Balloons. Three of my colleagues had been the masterminds. As one of them said, "No one should have to have chemotherapy on Valentine's Day."

My planning period was first thing in the morning, and I had a chance to truly sit in this moment. Valentine after valentine. It was incredible.

< 124 >

Jason: *Beth sent me pictures of all the cards she had received, all covering her desk. I have to admit, I got a teary-eyed as I sat in my office. To think of all the people who had taken part in this…it was overwhelming. And I know it meant the world to Beth.*

Beth: Fourth period arrived quickly, and that meant the return to the Cancer Center. At least this time, I knew what to expect. I remember wondering on my drive how it must feel for the infusion nurses knowing that the first time they meet a patient, the patient looks completely normal. Then, upon the return for the second treatment, in most cases, there is a stark difference in appearance - no hair. It made me really sad for them.

Jason met me in the lobby, and we waited to be taken back.

This week's appointment was with the nurse practitioner at the Cancer Care Center. I quickly fell in love with her. You can't not do so. She is a blonde ball of energy. She went through my blood counts and called me a "model patient." This was important because if my counts were too low, I could not have my next round of chemotherapy. Quickly, we wrapped up the appointment, and she led me back to the fish tank waiting room.

The infusion nurse came out through the locked door of the chemotherapy suite and brought me to the room closest to the window. It was awesome to be able to see trees while getting an infusion cocktail that I knew would make me sick later. Fortunately, with the cocktail I was on, side effects did not increase. If you did not have terrible side effects the first time, you likely would not have them for the next infusions.

Jason and I sat together while the drugs ran through my veins. I showed him the valentines from the kids, and we watched a movie.

< 125 >

Midway through the infusion, the nurse asked Jason his plans for Valentine's Day. She point-blank asked if he had something planned. Jason's face tried to hide it, but I could tell he had something planned at home.

Upon finishing, I drove myself home, and to my "surprise," Jason had roses (which are my favorite), chocolate, and dinner ready for us. It was perfect. Chemotherapy on Valentine's Day ended up not being too terrible.

I went back to work Friday, and then we had a long weekend for Presidents' Day. On Tuesday, the day I was supposed to go back to work, I couldn't get out of bed. First, we thought I was running a fever, then we thought maybe a stomach virus, but I didn't have any symptoms. My body had just given up, and it was taking everything I had for Harper. It was the first and only unplanned day that I took off school. I just couldn't do it. We never figured out what happened.

The rest of the month was filled with baby appointments. When I suffered my miscarriage in April, I had found out that I have a uterine abnormality.

My uterus is slightly heart-shaped. Because of that, there is a slight risk of preterm labor. That meant every two weeks from week 22-28, I would need cervical ultrasounds to check and make sure that Harper was not coming early. At 28 weeks, the likelihood of her survival went through the roof.

Jason: *On an intellectual level, I understood we were having a baby. But there were times it still didn't feel quite real yet, that something might go wrong again.*

< 126 >

I didn't dwell on these feelings and pushed them out of my mind when they popped in. But every time Beth didn't feel right, every time she said she hadn't felt Harper kick in a little while, there was that fear that it could happen again. And the thought of that was almost too much to bear.

Beth: Each ultrasound I had confirmed that things looked great. The only thing that the doctor noticed was that Harper's kidney was not emptying properly. It was an issue that we were told they would watch, but it could resolve itself. If not, Harper would be evaluated by a pediatric urologist at birth.

The month slipped by quickly, which meant the third trimester and Harper's delivery were fast approaching.

< 127 >

< 128 >

11. 2 YEARS

Beth: March brought a (relative) feeling of normalcy.

Time seemed to fall into two spaces - doctors' appointments and the time waiting to go doctors' appointments. If it was not a chemotherapy appointment, it was for Harper - glucose testing (twice - failed the first one), ultrasounds, and regular checkups. We finally reached the 3rd trimester - a blessing, but it also meant appointments every single week.

Thankfully, everything looked great on all accounts - Harper was growing just as she should. My cervical ultrasounds every two weeks ceased.

With all that was happening, Jason and I almost forgot one important date.

Our anniversary. On March 11, we would celebrate two years of marriage.

I innocently asked Jason where he would want to go, and his response was..

"I don't care."

We ended up going back to the Melting Pot, which is a favorite of ours. The year before, we had rose petals on our table, a 1st anniversary sign, and candles too. We ate and drank a lot of wine that night... and then, a week later, a positive pregnancy test.

This year was different.

< 129 >

We were expecting another baby... but not the same baby as on that pregnancy test.

I spent an hour crying in front of the mirror. I couldn't find a dress to wear to dinner that matched a headscarf. Then, I couldn't wear the dress I wanted because the prosthesis would not fit into the bra I needed to wear.

As I put makeup on, I just stared.

My face was not mine. It looks puffy and red from the steroids. I just had chemotherapy the week before, and I looked sick.

Red. Bald. Puffy. Gross.

The dress I found to wear had stains from lotion that kept my skin's dryness under control. I just didn't care.

The only thing that looked beautiful was my round belly.

That beautiful little girl who loved to kick and her kicks were perfection.

When we arrived at the Melting Pot, the contrast to the year before was so clear. This year, we were in a tiny corner of the restaurant in a tiny corner seat (that my belly barely fit into). The waiter barely paid attention to us. There was also no wine.

However, it was perfect.

Jason: *The contrast to the same meal at the same restaurant one year earlier was stark. Not that we didn't take joy in celebrating our anniversary, but it also felt like we had lived 10 lifetimes in the last 365 days. It was an odd feeling to take stock of just how much our lives had changed since the last time we walked into that restaurant. It also made me wonder how many things could change in the next year.*

< 130 >

Would we come back in 2020 and marvel at how crazy our lives still were compared to now?

Would we even have that opportunity?

Beth: Jason and I had barely a moment to breathe. Every "special occasion" was marred with anxiety and anticipation.

This was the first time that we could celebrate. Celebrate two years of marriage and come 10 weeks from now, we would be holding the miracle that we had prayed for in our arms.

The next week, I had an appointment with the maternal fetal medicine specialist. I had not been to see since Harper's anatomy scan, and it had taken FOREVER to get an appointment with her. It took multiple emails and phone calls from myself and the high-risk OB at my OB/GYN.

The sole reason to see her was to double check my starting a new chemotherapy, Taxol. We also wanted to confirm my delivery date.

The MFM came in and smiled at me.

"You making it? How are you feeling?"

"Very pregnant."

That was my standard answer. Saying that my throat was on fire, and I felt gross and fat probably would be frowned upon.

She read through my file and looked at the oncologist's plan moving forward. Taxol with Herceptin and Perjeta after delivery.

"My recommendation is delivery at 34 weeks."

< 131 >

Wait. What? I must have not heard her right.

> "You can't have these targeted drugs while you are pregnant, and that is a big deal. We should deliver the baby early. It would be in your best interest."

"Wouldn't that mean she would need to be in the NICU?"

She said yes and talked about how we would be able to tour the NICU prior to giving birth.

That was not much of a comfort.

As she talked, I could feel my stomach knotting... again and again and again. I felt the tears.

> Both of our nephews had spent time in the NICU, so I had a relatively sound understanding of what a delivery at 34 weeks meant and everything it encompassed.

> Harrison, our oldest nephew, was a 34-weeker. He was in the NICU for two weeks before being able to come home. Obviously, Griffin had also faced substantial health issues right after birth.

> I could not stop thinking about the risk for Harper... the fact that she would not be coming home with us right away. After going through surgeries and treatment after treatment, I couldn't even bring home my baby? That couldn't be normal after all we had been through?

> Not once did the oncologist seem concerned about not starting the targeted treatment right away. Communication between medical professionals broke down for the first time.

< 132 >

I began to cry. There was not anything else to do except cry. Jason was not there. It was just me.

The MFM said she could call my OB/GYN and oncologist and tell them the plan. I nodded yes absentmindedly. My mind was not wrapping around what was happening. The MFM gave me a pat on the back and told me that I would get through this.

I walked out of that office as quickly as I could.

The elevator ride down was a blur.... There were tears. A lot of tears.

After making it to the atrium, I sat down and called Jason. He was on his way to Pittsburgh for work. He was going to be gone for two days.

After one ring, he answered. I could not even get out hello.

"They want to deliver Harper at 34 weeks. That means the end of April."

Jason: *I was stunned. This was the first we had even heard about the potential for an early delivery. And with no discussion, it seemed already determined for us. The thought of not being able to take Harper home from the hospital right away was not something I could allow my mind to fathom. Not after everything else that had happened.*

Trying to process all of this behind the wheel of my rental car, some 200 miles from home, was brutal. I knew Beth needed me to be there, but even if I was able to cancel my work trip, I wouldn't pull into our driveway for close to four hours. At that moment, I felt about as helpless as I had at any point during this journey.

< 133 >

Beth: I drove myself to school, but I could not focus. I called the high-risk OB nurse to explain what was going on. She said she would talk to my OB/GYN also and fill her in.

My department chair and I spoke during lunch. By "spoke," I mean I bawled my eyes out. We talked about dates and subs and how I would manage getting through one of our classes' assessments. She calmed me down and handed me tissues. I could not get over the fact that our daughter would not start her life in our arms. She would be alone in an incubator at the hospital for an unknown amount of time.

I made it home and fell into our guest bed. I felt Harper kick, and I just lost it.

I called Jason and then my mother-in-law, both reassuring me it would be okay. Harper would be fine.

St. Elizabeth is a Level III NICU, equipped to be with the sickest of babies. Children's Hospital in Cincinnati was 15 minutes away. We were so fortunate to have some of the best children's hospitals in the country in our backyard.

Then my cell phone rang... blocked number.

For some reason, I answered it. Maybe it was because Jason was out of town... maybe a feeling.

It was my oncologist. She asked me how I was doing. What a loaded question.

I sat on the carpet and could feel the tears welling in my eyes.

"Been better."

< 134 >

She told me she heard from the maternal fetal medicine specialist whom she had not been in contact with before. She asked about who she was and asked about the plan put in place.

The next words are ones that settled my heart.

"I had a 34-weeker, and it is terrible. We are going to talk about this."

She said she would keep in touch and hung up.

I laid on the floor alone and cried again. I called Jason to fill him in, and then headed to the grocery store to find something for dinner.

Within a minute of stepping into Kroger, my cell phone rang again. Unknown number.

I sat at the cafe in the Kroger Starbucks and answered.

"Hello?" It was the MFM from St. Elizabeth.

"Hi Beth, so I talked to your oncologist. She and I decided that 37 weeks is an appropriate time to deliver."

Her words took my breath away. I sat at Starbucks, stunned. What a turn of events in less than 12 hours.

"Are you sure?'

She said yes and good luck to us.

Immediately, I called Jason and could hear him holding back emotion. Relief. Pure relief. Our little girl would come at term and likely not need a single moment in the NICU.

< 135 >

Jason: *That day reinforced two things very clearly in my mind...we were incredibly lucky to have such amazing doctors who truly cared about us, and we really had very little control over anything at this point.*

We could do everything right, follow every doctor's order down to the letter, plan every last detail...and still get blindsided at any point. In hindsight, it was great training in learning to parent. Sometimes, there's absolutely nothing you can do but ride the wave and just hope you end up on your feet at the end.

Beth: The following week marked two significant milestones. First, it was Cincinnati's hometown holiday, Reds' opening day. I struggled to pull my only Cincinnati Reds shirt over my enormous belly.

Second, this would be my last Adriamycin and Cytoxan chemotherapy. I had made through twelve weeks of what they consider the harshest chemotherapy regimen for breast cancer. I had done so with minimal side effects (hair loss and heartburn) and only missed one non-treatment day of work.

It felt pretty awesome.

Jason and I sat and talked and worked through the push of the "Red Devil" and the Cytoxan drip. It was the start of my spring break, which meant maternity pictures that next weekend. April would bring baby showers and family in preparation for Harper's late May arrival.

Four chemotherapy treatments down, 12 more to finish.

< 136 >

12. WAITING FOR HARPER

Beth: We had a tentative induction time.

> Harper would come around the third week of May at 37 weeks. Jason and I were so thankful that my oncologist stepped in with her input on that delivery... not only as a doctor but as a mother.

The wait was on.

> After much deliberation, I decided I wanted to do maternity pictures. It was again something typical that normal pregnant ladies look forward to doing. I yearned for those moments. This meant contacting our wedding photographer to arrange the shoot. This also meant telling someone outside of those we interact with in our daily lives about my cancer diagnosis.

I opted for a phone call as opposed to a text. Cancer while pregnant warrants that.

> We made small talk for a few minutes, talking about kids and school. She knew I was pregnant, so we talked about how I was feeling and if I was getting excited.

Then, the question.

"Would you be willing to do a mini-maternity session for me?"

No hesitation in her response.

< 137 >

"Of course!"

She immediately started talking details. I let her finish and paused. I could feel myself turning red, a common occurrence when I feel insanely uncomfortable.

Initiate bombshell drop.

"I thought you would need to know that I have been going through breast cancer treatment, and I would like to do some pictures with me bald."

An audible pause.

"Okay. We can do this..."

The rest of the conversation was a blur.

We set the pictures on April 3 at Alms Park in Cincinnati, which happened to be the same place Jason and I did our wedding pictures. It is gorgeous, and it has some beautiful places to get great shots.

For these, I decided I wanted to get my makeup done since, for obvious reasons, I could not do my hair. I was incredibly excited to do a little pampering.

Jason: *She had been wavering about whether to get maternity pictures for a while. I wanted her to do it, but I also knew I wanted it to be a decision she reached by herself and was comfortable with. I knew she would want them one day; after all, the point is to capture the journey. And though our journey was a little different than most, that's what made it special.*

< 138 >

I know it wasn't easy for her, and I know it took a ton of courage for her to be comfortable enough to take the pictures with no hair, but I was proud she did it.

Beth: When I arrived for my appointment at Ulta Beauty, I almost turned around and drove home. As I sat in my car, I felt like I was going to die. The fear of running into someone I knew, someone who did not know I had cancer, someone who just stared at the noticeable pregnant belly and lack of hair. I was paralyzed in fear.

I opened the car door and got out. For the two minutes it took to go from the car to the store, I ducked my head and waddled as quickly as I could. This continued even as I made my way to the back of the store to the beauty salon.

As a high school teacher, I know that my teenage students frequent Ulta Beauty. To see them in this moment - raw, anxious, and uncomfortable - would be awful. My facade as a positive cancer fighter would be shattered. I was not ready for that wall to come down... for my students to see me in that most vulnerable state.

The cashier at the salon introduced me to my makeup artist for the appointment, and together, we picked out some fun eye makeup colors. I had not had my makeup done since our wedding two years ago, so it was a lot of fun.

As she did my makeup, the artist asked questions, and I responded genuinely. You could tell she did not want to address the elephant in the room, but at this point, I was used to that.

< 139 >

About midway through my appointment, the makeup artist asked me to take my headscarf off. She wanted to innocently blend the makeup line between my headscarf and my face. I whipped my head around, investigating and analyzing who was around me.

Initially, I heard myself say no. I took a breath and slipped the scarf off my head.

My heart pounded for what seemed like an hour - it was only about three minutes.

And it was done. I paid for the makeup and slid out of there as unassumingly as possible.

Later that evening, I slipped on a lavender maternity dress and a navy, pink, and lavender headscarf. The dress hugged my belly in a way that was beautiful. Feeling and seeing Harper move in my stomach was incredible but seeing this belly was something spectacular. With all that was happening, there were a few moments that I truly took the time to savor that this little person was growing inside of me.

I met the photographer, and although it was a chilly April evening, it was beautiful. It reminded me of the atmosphere the night we were married. A slight chilled wind during the golden hour.

At Alms Park, there is a stone pavilion with both covered and uncovered spaces. That was our first stop.

The photographer had me pose in different positions - sitting, standing, leaning. Me holding my belly and looking down at it. Me holding my belly and smiling at the camera.

Typical maternity photos.

Perfect first-time mom moments.

< 140 >

After about 10 minutes, she looked at me.

"Want to do a few without your head scarf?"

>I had prepared for this moment. This is why I wanted to do the maternity photos in the first place. I wanted Harper to see that years from now what we did together. What we made it through together.

Briefly in that split-second, I felt shame. Shame for my baldness.

And then off came the headscarf.

Snap. Snap. Snap.

>We moved from one location on the pavilion to an overlook next to the Ohio River. Some of our favorite wedding pictures were taken there. It is breathtaking.

I brought a onesie that had been given to us by our friends who had introduced us.

It was white with a pink ribbon on it.

It read: "My mom is my hero."

>With my bald head glistening in all of its glory and a perfect sunset in the background, I held it up for the camera.

CLICK.

>We finished the session, and I thanked her profusely. Before she left, the photographer asked about "sneak peeks." Typically, she would put a few on her Facebook prior to finishing the whole session. Given the sensitive nature of this, she promised to email me first with a few and wait for permission to post them publicly.

< 141 >

The next few days were quiet. I was on my three-week break from chemotherapy, gearing up for a new drug - Taxol - to begin in the middle of April. Baby showers were also coming - one from my amazing friends and Judi, and then a virtual shower from Jason's family. Spring Break truly allowed for some time to just be lazy and recuperate.

A ding into my inbox came on Friday.

My maternity pictures.

I opened the email and instantly cried.

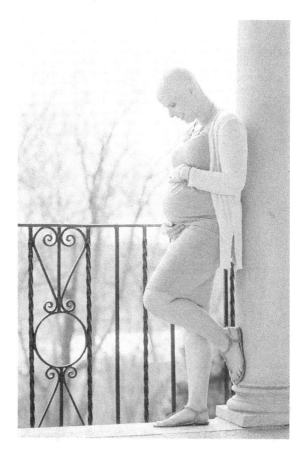

< 142 >

Every single photo was absolutely beautiful. Even bald. The lighting was perfect. The background was perfect. As awkward and self-conscious as I felt during so many of those shots, the photos instead showed an incredible confidence. I sat in our bedroom in one of my favorite chairs in our house - a beige armchair that we had gotten while still in our starter home.

Jason: *The pictures were amazing. Simply amazing. It seemed that each picture perfectly captured the myriad emotions and events that had overtaken our lives. And I knew that these pictures, with her being bald, were going to tell a powerful story to our daughter. A story of what her mom went through, and overcame. To me, there was nothing more powerful than that message.*

Beth: I took a breath and knew that I wanted to share these with everyone. It had taken seven months, but I was ready to let people into our world. I wanted a chance to share our joy.

I selected one picture. It was me against a pillar at the pavilion at Alms Park. The golden hour sun glistened in the background. It illuminated my very pregnant body - bringing out the lavender in my dress and the shine of my bald head. It slightly washed out my profile, but it brought attention to me staring down at my stomach.

The moment glowed.

I took a breath and wrote down what I wanted to share.

What a journey it has been to this moment. Tomorrow marks 31 weeks - 6 weeks until we get to finally meet our little girl. To say the last seven months have been emotionally and physically challenging is an understatement. I have been back and forth about sharing this part of our journey - that

< 143 >

baby girl and I went through two surgeries and chemotherapy together to treat early-stage breast cancer during my pregnancy. However, both are so intertwined. Plus - everything looks so good - baby girl has been measuring on target (and MOVING like crazy) and my prognosis is CURATIVE (caught so early!) thanks to all of the doctors and nurses who have worked so hard to collaborate to make sure both of us were healthy and well-taken care of. I can't say enough about the OBs and nurses. There is still a way to go, but this picture captures my pregnancy perfectly. To those who supported the three of us from the beginning - our family - our absolute rock, friends, colleagues, and strangers who have prayed for us - thank you. This little girl is beyond loved. One thing I want to say - to my friends (yes - you in your 30s) - please be vigilant when doing self-breast exams. If something seems off, go to the doctor. Trust your gut.

I read it so many times before putting out into the social media sphere. Another weight off my shoulders. I could now share more joy and hope for others. I could make good on the promise that Jason and I had made to God. The promise that we would share His miracles for us to show that He is amazing.

However, although there was so much happiness, I continued to feel a dark cloud forming in my head. Things that had not bothered me throughout my pregnancy and treatments began to make me feel out of control.

Food became my trigger.

People who know me understand that I have a deep love for food. I love to cook and to eat. I love trying new restaurants. My OB/GYN, thankfully, was awesome about being specific about what I could not eat. Honestly, there was not a lot at all. There were the obvious ones - no soft

< 144 >

unpasteurized cheese, lunch meats, and alcohol. Otherwise, that was it. As for with cancer treatments, the nurse navigator told me to eat what I could

However, over Spring Break, a moment threw me over a precipice. Jason had to get his bumper repaired because of a mishap while we were in Gatlinburg for our babymoon. For most of Spring Break, I dropped him off at work. It was near a great smoothie place in an area called Oakley. I felt great as I was on my chemotherapy break for three weeks. I stopped there and ordered a peanut butter and banana smoothie. Instead of stevia, the cashier added a little of raw honey. It was tasty and a welcome treat for a pregnant woman.

As I sat in the car drinking my smoothie, my mind wandered to the use of the raw honey. On the drive home, I decided to call the place to confirm that was an ingredient used. She affirmed it came from a farm in Ohio and hung up.

I am not sure why, but I began Googling if pregnant women can eat raw honey.

I came across something about not pregnant women but cancer patients. Raw honey can make cancer patients ill because of us being immunocompromised.

Trying to be sensible, I called the nurse navigator at the Cancer Center. In the four months of treatment, I called maybe once or twice. My favorite nurse navigator was not in that day, so I left a message for the one in the office.

Some time passed, and the cancer center number popped up on my phone.

"Hello?"

< 145 >

The nurse navigator introduced herself and restated my question about the raw honey. She said directly not to let that happen again while going through chemotherapy. She explained why, but I did not hear her. I was on the verge of a panic attack.

After we hung up, I almost threw up.

Actually, I dry heaved into our kitchen trash can.

That moment changed my relationship with food permanently.

Every crumb of food that I put into my mouth became a constant onslaught of fear.

What if this is not pasteurized?

What if it was not stored properly and I get Listeria?

What if I eat something that hurts Harper?

The anxiety left me frozen in fear.

> **Jason:** *Though I'm not an anxious person, her food anxiety started to wear off on me. Every time I stopped on the way home from work to pick up dinner, or ran to the store to stock up on groceries, I found myself double-checking labels, asking questions, Googling ingredients....you name it. Food was always something I put minimal thought into; now it was becoming like a part-time job to find something we could feel comfortable eating.*
>
> *I wondered if this was going to be like this forever for us. Would there ever again be a time where we could just go out to eat wherever we wanted, order whatever we wanted, and not give it a second thought?*
>
> **Beth:** *The emails I sent to the high-risk OB nurse were always about food. The fear quickly became consuming. She called it "Pregnancy Anxiety,"*

< 146 >

and in conversation with my OB/GYN, it comes from a place of wanting to protect the child. The doctor warned me that this could be an issue even after delivery. We would need to monitor it very closely.

Even with the anxiety, moments of joy found their way while we waited for Harper's arrival.

Baby showers.

Two of my best friends and Judi put the first one on. My friend hosted it at her beautiful house, and it was Disney themed - just like Harper's nursery. It had my favorite foods - tacos, a watermelon that looked like a Mickey head, and mimosas that I couldn't partake in.

I hired a student of mine who was interested in culinary arts to bake and decorate cupcakes for the event. They were absolutely perfect - lavender icing complete with a glitter crown on top.

We played Disney-themed games and just enjoyed each other's company. What more could you truly ask for? Friends and family there to celebrate the miracle in our life. Although there were moments that my anxiety made itself known (thinking about every single thing I ate and drank), I felt immense joy.

After I opened gifts, I just looked around at each face in the room.

All I could think about is that this tribe of women - all from different moments of my life (high school, college, work, and adulthood) - made the entire experience that much easier. These were the women whom I would have been lost without. The women whom I always strived to be like. My role models.

< 147 >

The high from the weekend brought us to a significant moment on my chemotherapy journey.

That Thursday, I started Taxol.

Initially, I was supposed to be done with chemotherapy after I finished Adriamycin and Cytoxan until I delivered Harper. However, my oncologist thought we could squeeze in two more treatments of Taxol prior to delivery. The more treatments, the better the chance to ensure the cancer was gone.

After Harper's delivery, I would begin Herceptin and Perjeta, two drugs that are specific to HER2+ Breast Cancer. Those were the same two drugs that led to the heated discussion about my delivery date.

Taxol was very different because it was not nearly as toxic as the Adriamycin and Cytoxan. Those are the heavy hitters and wipe out EVERYTHING. Taxol, especially on a weekly basis, does not cause nausea and the debilitating fatigue.

When Jason and I arrived, we met with the oncologist and talked about my final official delivery date. She assured me that this chemotherapy regimen would not be nearly as awful as the last. To put in perspective, Jason could touch the utensils I used as opposed to when I did the AC chemo.

When I sat down in the familiar chemotherapy chair, the infusion nurse talked a little bit about my pre-medication. Taxol, derived from Pacific Yew tree bark, can cause severe allergic reactions. For this chemotherapy and here on, after going through the 12 rounds, I would receive IV Benadryl.

< 148 >

As she pushed the Benadryl, Jason showed me an article that I could read. During my other four treatments, I did schoolwork and puzzles with Jason with no issue.

And then the IV Benny (as it is affectionately called) hit my system.

HARD.

I could not keep my eyes open. I felt DRUNK. It felt like my 21st birthday all over again... when I was kicked out of two bars for passing out.

The nurse came in and turned off the lights.

I fell asleep.

I groggily woke up for a few minutes to hear the infusion nurse explain how the Taxol drip would run.

The first one would be longer than the rest because of the risk of having an allergic reaction. After each 15-minute interval, they would increase the speed of the infusion.

All went well. No allergic reaction. Instead of 90 minutes, the next 11 would only be an hour.

Eleven. It was hard to conceptualize even making it through 11 more treatments.

I went home and laid down. That was the chemotherapy routine. However, the next morning, I felt normal. It was a welcome change from the last 12 weeks.

That weekend, Jason's family threw a virtual shower for us. With family spread out all over the country - from Minnesota to Florida, Jason's mom,

< 149 >

sister, and aunt planned this for us. Our families sent gifts to our house, and on the day of the shower, we would open them together and get a lot of pictures.

Fortunately, I felt pretty great for that shower. There would have been NO WAY I could have functioned through it on Adriamycin and Cytoxan. I wore my favorite headscarf - the one I had from my maternity pictures and the shower the week prior to this. I pulled on a lavender tunic that showed my 33-week bump just perfectly.

Jason's mom and sister shooed us out of the house for a few hours. It was glorious to just go have lunch and relax. Upon our return, the house was decked out in lavender balloons, along with a silver set spelling out Harper's name. The cake was Mickey and Winnie-the-Pooh themed, complete with Disney figurines that Harper could eventually play with.

The weather was absolutely perfect for April - no rain and warm temperatures.

It was wonderful. A perfect Easter Sunday.

This following week brought such excitement that it went so slowly. It would be my last chemotherapy session prior to Harper being born. For months, it felt like this moment would never arrive.

The giddy feeling intensified as I walked into the infusion room. In honor of the day, I brought cookies and thank-you notes. Although there were still 10 to go, we had prayed for this moment. I was 34 weeks pregnant, Harper was healthy, and my body had withstood the toxic treatments.

When my oncologist walked back into the infusion room to see Jason and me, she opened the curtain with a huge smile on her face. The mood was entirely different from the previous appointments.

< 150 >

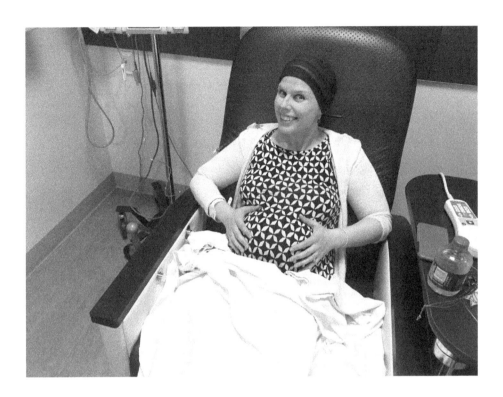

"This is it!"

She did her exam, checking for neuropathy and swelling. All checked out to be perfect. Many people ice their fingers and toes during Taxol to stop the chemotherapy from ravaging the nerve endings. So far, all had been amazing.

She showed me how she had Harper's delivery date in her phone, and her goal was to stop by while I was in the hospital to meet Harper.

There were so many tears in that exam room. I could tell that there was a sense of relief on my oncologist's end. Her face said it. Her eyes said it. I cannot imagine how scary it is to not only worry about the health of the

< 151 >

actual cancer patient but the other patient there too. This was a joyous moment for everyone. We had made it.

Then, IV Benny kicked in, and I slept through most of the infusion.

The month ended with a "Nacho average baby shower" thrown by our English department. There were tacos to be had and margaritas for everyone else. It was an incredible way to celebrate the end of April and prepare for Harper's birth month.

< 152 >

13. DAR LA LUZ (BIRTH)

Beth: "She is out!"

Time stopped. Life changed.

Again.

The month, until that moment, seemed to drag on. It was the first month in 2019 that I had not sat in an infusion chair or seen my oncologist.

May brought final doctors' appointments, non-stress tests, and ultrasounds. It looked like Harper would be about six pounds at birth. Considering babies exposed to chemotherapy tend to be small, in addition to my food anxiety during my third trimester, we counted our blessings that she would be somewhat average.

We finished Harper's room on Mother's Day. That day brought a myriad of feelings. On Mother's Day 2018, Griffin almost died. On Mother's Day 2018, I did not know if I was truly a mother or not after our miscarriage. Mother's Day 2019, we were two weeks away from welcoming Harper. I dealt with the question: was Harper making me a mother, or was I already one?

And for the last nine months, I had held my breath.

< 153 >

Jason: *There's really no good way to describe the emotions you feel as you prepare for your first child. Which, in itself, is actually kind of odd because becoming a parent is a pretty common thing. So why can no one really do it justice in words?*

Maybe it's because you just have to experience it. Everyone always gives you advice, tells you how much things will change and, how different your life will be. But it really is hard to grasp the enormity of how true those statements are until you're in the hospital room, looking at a tiny baby and knowing that you're responsible for her life. You're no longer the guy who wears the same basketball shorts for days, tilts chip bags to eat crumbs, or can name every Florida football player but not all the Supreme Court Justices.

Now you're Dad. Now you have to get it together, and keep it together, because it's not about you anymore. It's about her. And though that responsibility is colossal, you'll come to realize it's the best thing you'll ever do.

For years, whenever Beth and I talked about having kids, I worried about a lot of things. Could I financially support a family? Could I be a good role model? Would I be able to instill the right values in a kid? I even worried about whether I could help a kid with their homework past a certain age. If you saw my grades in high school, you'd probably question that too.

Beth: A cry.

I did not care what it took to get there - the number of doctors' appointments, more trips to labor and delivery than worth counting, toxic chemicals pumping through my veins, and sleepless nights on the couch.

< 154 >

I just wanted to hear crying. A cry.

A moment of silence after the OB/GYN's announcement.

And then wailing. More like screaming.

I have never felt that immense amount of joy, relief, and fear in my entire life.

My first words:

"Does she sound normal?!"

> Looking back, those are not quite the words I wanted to use, but I had been so scared for so long that I could not relax until I asked.

"Yes," my OB/GYN replied, smiling.

After nine long months, I remembered how to breathe.

The 17 hours leading up to this moment had not been without some excitement.

> Jason and I arrived at the hospital at 7:00 a.m. on Monday, May 20. We chose it because it would put Harper at "term" for her birth. She would not be considered premature and likely would not have the complications that could come with early delivery. This, again, was thanks to my oncologist speaking out against an earlier delivery. I also chose this date because of the OB/GYN. Because of being high risk, I saw every single OB/GYN in the practice. All of them were fabulous, but I had a few favorites. One of them was on call that day.

God does not make mistakes. This doctor was meant to see the completion of the miracle.

< 155 >

Jason: *I always feared that I would be one of those dads who was driving his wife to the hospital at 2:00 a.m., speeding through red lights to make sure we got there in time (and avoiding the biggest fear...having to deliver the child myself in the backseat of the car on the side of the road).*

But even with that off the table, I was admittedly still nervous. And excited. And anxious. And a whole lot of feelings that I couldn't put into words. Because even though we had cleared all of the pre-parenting rites of passage, with baby showers and painting the nursery and loading up on diapers, I'm still not sure either of us fully grasped what was coming.

I just remember having a strange feeling as I backed out of the garage that morning, knowing that when we pulled back into it in a couple days, we would have a baby girl with us.

Beth: After arriving, they took us to our room.

It was HUGE in terms of size, but even more importantly, it was an incredibly warm space. It had huge windows, beautiful wall paneling, and a nice painting above the bed. If it was the room we would be in for the long haul, I was totally okay with this.

Before long, a nurse walked in. She had such a wonderful aura around her, like a young grandmother. She introduced herself and said she would be there until 7:00 p.m. that evening.

It quickly dawned on me that I had heard her name before. I quickly texted my very close friend and asked her the name of the nurse who had been with her through her deliveries.

By coincidence, it was the same nurse.

< 156 >

Except Jason and I came to realize through all of this that coincidences do not exist.

When she returned, I told her who my friend was. She grinned.

I also told her that when my friend told the stories about the deliveries of her three children, she always mentioned how much of a blessing she was.

I knew at that moment that on this day, on the day our daughter was born, we were truly in the best hands.

We went through the obligatory "delivery" things - bloodwork, drug testing, and vitals. My oncologist had fortunately given the thumbs up to use my port, so I would not have IVs in my hands/arm during delivery. It would be far more comfortable during the whole labor part.

Then we waited.

And waited.

Eventually, the nurse came in to start the Pitocin in order to kick start the whole process. More waiting.

There was a steady stream of people to come in and check on me. My OB/GYN's office was attached to the hospital, so one of the doctors came over and said hi. He told me he saw my name on the schedule and wanted to see if I needed anything. He did this after being in surgery. I will say this forever. That practice has the most caring group of doctors.

Jason: *A half-dozen different nurses and doctors popped in, making sure Beth was comfortable, checking her vitals, measuring the baby's vitals, and doing a lot of other things that I had no clue about. But as the morning slowly morphed into afternoon, we still didn't appear to be too much closer to having a baby.*

< 157 >

I was also getting continually uneasy at the comments being made by the nurses and doctors as they bounced around the room. Comments that referred to my involvement with the birth, where I would stand, how I would be assisting. Perhaps they thought I was a doctor? Short of that, I'm not sure why my role continued to be a topic of conversation (much to Beth's delight). I wasn't sure how well I was going to handle being in the same room when she gave birth, let alone being involved in the action.

Beth: Then, the high-risk OB nurse came in - our incredible angel. She delivered four simple words.

"You can do this."

One last bit of her encouragement and wisdom.

She told me she had my OB/GYN on speed dial and would expect updates from him throughout the day. I was so grateful to see her face because of all she had done for our family. She truly served as the liaison between my oncologist, the OB/GYN office, and the maternal fetal medicine specialist. There had been few moments that I ever felt things were not streamlined. In large part, it was because of her.

That was really the extent of the day. Eventually, I received the amazing thing in labor... the epidural. It allowed me to relax a little bit more.

And continued waiting... and many, many red Popsicles.

And watching the Amazing Race - Season 1.

About mid-afternoon, I noticed on the monitor that Harper's heart rate changed. The nurse taught us what it should like.

"Steady humps - no dips."

< 158 >

Immediately, I called for her and began to hyperventilate. She handed me an oxygen mask and put a washcloth on my face. Jason held my hand. The nurse tried to position me in order to help Harper's heart rate. She began to stabilize.

That is when my OB/GYN came in with the most serious look on his face thus far. That is saying something, considering what I had been through.

"I am not trying to say this to scare you. But if this happens again, we are going to have to talk about a C-section."

I looked at Jason and said,

"Okay. That's okay. That means I do not have to take two weeks unpaid."

Obviously, I was delirious and terrified.

Jason: *His tone was measured, but he made it clear that the situation could deteriorate rapidly and if that happened, they were going to have to act fast. All of a sudden, being bored in the hospital room was the least of my worries. What if something went wrong in the birth? We hadn't even met her yet but already we were being apprised of potential problems. Talk about feeling helpless.*

It was definitely our first "welcome to being a parent" moment.

Beth: "If that happens, I will not come in and explain it. I am explaining it now. We will need to move quickly at that point," he continued.

I realized at that moment that we could be talking about a life-or-death situation for Harper. I kept breathing into the mask.

< 159 >

He paused and reassured us that no matter what, all would be fine.

Our nurse and the OB put in an internal monitor for Harper to keep an even closer eye on her heart rate.

After that, I refused to move. I was convinced that if I moved, Harper could die.

Hours passed.

When the time reached 7:00 p.m., it was time for a nurse shift change. This meant that our labor and delivery angel would leave without meeting Harper. She promised to stop by the next day.

We met our next nurse, who was also fabulous.

More waiting.

At about 9:30 p.m., the nurse encouraged me to switch positions. She promised to keep an eye on the monitor.

We did, and Harper was fine - steady heart rate.

More time passed... and then, we noticed changes on the monitor.

It was "go time."

My OB/GYN joked that he had two mothers racing to have a baby first that night.

Harper lost. We thought we were going to have a May 20th birthday.

However, as with everything, Harper tends to do things in her own time. Harper Jaye Brubaker was born at 12:29 am on Tuesday, May 21, 2019. She weighed 5lbs, 4oz (an entire pound less than the ultrasound predicted) and measured 18.5 inches long.

< 160 >

My "normal sounding" baby was laid on my bare chest... on my mastectomy side. Again, not a coincidence. She made up for what I was missing... not only physically, but as a person.

Jason: *Hearing Harper cry for the first time, seeing Beth hold her...they were moments I will never forget. Everything else in our lives melted out of my mind. The only thing that mattered now was that little girl.*

Beth: Prior to Harper's delivery, Jason decided not to be the one to cut the umbilical cord. I was surprised when my OB/GYN asked if I wanted to do it.

"YES."

What a moment. Harper became her own person, not reliant on anyone else. That, in and of itself, was beautiful.

They moved us to our new room at about 2:30 am. Bless Jason's parents and my brother, who stayed until we were moved. That night, I could not sleep. I just kept staring at her. It had not sunk in that Harper was here. Months of anticipation and she was here. Healthy. No NICU time. Perfection.

The morning became a revolving door with our family and friends. It was wonderful to show our miracle to the world. We also had our wonderful photographer who has captured so many moments for us (the same one who did my maternity pictures) come do a "Fresh 48" session.

Harper had made it. We had made it.

< 161 >

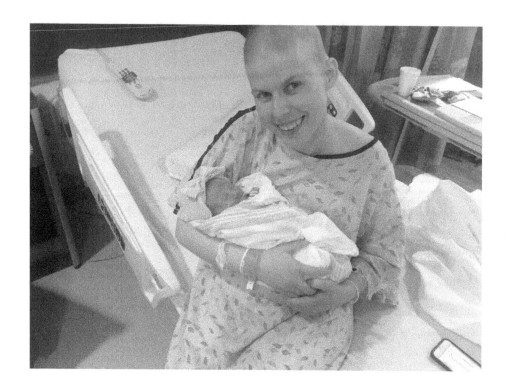

Jason: *The whole time in the hospital felt surreal, but in a wonderful way. We had waited and hoped and prayed for this moment, and when it arrived, we were overwhelmed with emotion. Knowing that this little girl was here, knowing that this was our new family...it was amazing.*

Beth: The next day, we waited for discharge. We met one pediatrician in the practice we had chosen for Harper, and he gave her a clean bill of health. The wait was then for my OB/GYN.

When he came, he reminded us (with his incredibly dry sense of humor) that not being able to breastfeed was perfectly fine.

"Just stare into her eyes when you feed her. There is the emotional attachment."

< 162 >

I appreciated so much about him. It was also not lost on Jason or me that this was the doctor in whose office we heard that there was no heartbeat for our son.

Now, 13 months later, he was sending us home with our daughter.

> **Jason:** *Talk about a sign from above. From delivering the worst possible news we could hear in that moment to, a little over a year later, telling us we were ready to take our daughter home. This was no coincidence.*
>
> *Even in our exhausted and sleep-deprived state, we recognized how special that moment was.*

Beth: Jason's parents fortunately stayed with us for the week to help us. They were fantastic.

> When you are sent home with a baby, there is no instruction manual. They wheel you out of the hospital and send you on your way.

Needless to say, Jason and I were terrified. The first night was ROUGH.

> The bassinet we had for Harper swallowed her up, and she kept rolling on her side. Everything you read is that a baby should always be on their back - "back is best" is on all of the sleep sacks.
>
> Well, her rolling on her side freaked us out to no end. (Babies just roll on their sides - they are fine. Again, we just had no experience). We basically held Harper all night.
>
> The next morning, without hesitation, we handed Harper to Jason's parents and went to Target to find a new bassinet.

As we pulled away, Jason looked me in the eye and said,

< 163 >

"We could just go to a hotel for an hour and sleep."

> **Jason:** *I was only half-joking. At that moment, I would have gladly paid any amount of money for just an hour of uninterrupted sleep.*

Beth: There is no type of tired like new parent tired.

We found a bassinet, and the next night was a little better.

> Jason's parents stayed through the weekend, and before they left, Jason's mom presented me with a beautiful book of pictures from each of my first six chemotherapy treatments. Jason had always been very secretive about the photos he took during my treatments. I found out it was because he was sending them to his mom.

> When she handed it to me, I bawled. So many emotions. The last page was a picture she had taken just a day or two ago - a picture of the three of us with Harper wearing a onesie that Jason gave me for Christmas.

It read: "My mom kicked cancer's butt."

It was perfection. Another reminder of how much we had been through.

Jason's parents left that Monday, and we began to settle in a routine (ish).

> The routine was not sleeping, feeding on demand, and endless blowouts. There were so many cute (and soiled) onesies.

> **Jason:** *The first week was - to put it mildly - rough. As I'm sure it is for all new parents. Your entire life is suddenly flipped upside down as you realize that a tiny baby now is in complete control.*

> *That's why you find yourself trying to keep your composure as you attempt to re-swaddle your daughter at 3:00 a.m. in the dark, without*

< 164 >

contacts, and trying to do so quietly to allow your wife to keep sleeping... only to have her pop her arm out of the blanket just as you're laying her back in the bassinet.

Or trying to avoid swearing profusely when, a few seconds after putting a fresh diaper on her, you immediately hear the unmistakable sound of a blowout.

Or, late on a weeknight, you find yourself wandering the unfamiliar baby section of a store, head down, mumbling to yourself like a crazy person, as you try to find the exact brand of wipes or diapers or formula that your wife tasked you with getting.

Or wondering how many baby spit-up stains are tolerated on a shirt before you should no longer wear it in public.

It was simultaneously exhausting and frustrating and eye-opening and humbling. But it was also wonderful. Being a parent, even with all the challenges, was a terrific feeling.

Beth: Harper had her one-week checkup, and that was our first introduction to our wonderful pediatrician. From the moment she picked Harper up, I knew that this woman needed to be Harper's doctor. Every movement during the exam was a snuggle and a show of love.

We found out later that both her mother and sister were breast cancer survivors. She understood what we were going through.

Harper had made it back to her birth weight, and the pediatrician said she looked great. Harper was still measuring in the 1% of height and weight. Because of Harper's kidney, we would have an ultrasound done at Children's Hospital in June.

< 165 >

One thing Harper's pediatrician mentioned was to be mindful about taking her out in public. Harper was relying on my antibodies until she had her first big set of vaccinations at eight weeks.

That sent me into a tailspin. I was terrified that Harper was going to get sick and die. The anxiety was stifling and began to really simmer after that.

On top of that, another thing was hanging over us. On May 30, I would return to the fateful infusion chair and begin chemotherapy yet again. This time, we would add two new drugs, Herceptin and Perjeta. The two drugs caused the disagreement about Harper's delivery date.

It would also be the first time that Jason could not go with me to one of my treatments.

At his urging, I asked one of my closest friends (the same friend who helped throw my baby shower) to come with me. Normally, my treatments took about two hours, including my doctor's appointment. My friend mentioned dinner plans, so no big deal. My appointment was at 11:00 a.m.

She picked me up, and off we went to the Cancer Care center.

The snowball effect started.

My doctor's appointment was running late (cancer time). My friend waited in the waiting room for me.

When my oncologist saw me, there were hugs and tears. She looked elated. We talked about Harper a lot.

She explained today I would start Herceptin and Perjeta. That would be every three weeks until next year. That would be on top of weekly Taxol for the next 10 weeks.

< 166 >

We talked about fertility. While I was pregnant, essentially, that pregnancy was protecting my ovaries from damage from the chemotherapy. That safety net was gone.

"Are you thinking you might want more children?"

Jason and I had gone into this pregnancy (and our miscarriage) with the idea that we would be "one and done." Maybe it was hormones, but I was not ready to shut the door on that quite yet.

I wanted a chance... so many chances had been taken. The chance to breastfeed... the chance to have a normal maternity leave.

"Yes... maybe?"

That meant we would add a monthly hormone suppression injection called Lupron. It goes right into your backside muscle, and the injection hurts like hell.

The oncologist then walked me back to the waiting room, and out quickly came one of the infusion nurses to come grab me. Upon entering the infusion room, all the nurses wanted to see Harper pictures. They fortunately got me the largest infusion room because it was a revolving door. Hope in a place that sometimes feels a little hopeless.

We sat down and one of the infusion nurses brought in my premeds.

IV Benny, Steroids, and Zofran... and Pepcid. No more liquid Pepcid (more awful taste ever) - just the pill form now.

While I was beginning to doze off, my oncologist came in with a gift bag.

"This is a little something for Harper."

< 167 >

Inside of the bag was a white-painted wooden placard with Harper's name on it. There was a heart next to her name. You could smell the wood had been engraved. A thoughtful gesture from not just a doctor, but another mother. From that day, it has sat on Harper's bookshelf - another reminder of one of her healthcare heroes.

After my premeds, we sat and talked... and waited. Usually, even if the pharmacy is behind, it would be maybe 30 extra minutes.

It was more like an hour and a half.

I finally asked one of the infusion nurses what was happening.

One of my drugs, Perjeta, had not been approved by insurance. They were waiting for an appeal. Perjeta... one of the lifeline drugs for HER2+ breast cancer.

That is health insurance. My doctor fortunately and quickly filed an appeal and was waiting for a response.

Another hour passed. The amount of guilt I felt for my friend to be there waiting for now three and a half hours was like an anvil weighing on my shoulders. The amount of guilt I felt that Jason was home alone with our nine-day-old daughter. The guilt I felt that I was not home snuggling Harper.

It was crushing to the soul.

Jason: *There was some guilt on my part – actually a fair amount – for not being able to be there with her physically. From the day of her diagnosis, I promised that I would be by her side through all of it; yet she was now in the hospital without me.*

< 168 >

It couldn't be helped – I had to watch Harper and we obviously couldn't bring her to the hospital. On an intellectual level, I recognized this was unavoidable and it wasn't anybody's fault. But I still felt some regret at not being able to live up to my promise to be there physically for everything.

Beth: Finally, after chicken salad sandwiches and some tears, my drugs were ready. For my first Herceptin and Perjeta, they had to be run slowly for an hour in case of an allergic reaction. Each one took an hour with 30 minutes in between.

I did not start my Taxol infusion until almost 4:00 p.m. Five hours and counting in the hospital.

After six hours, two new drugs, an insurance denial (and then approval), and a really painful hormone shot, we walked out of the Cancer Care center.

I apologized a million times to my friend. She had missed dinner with her former students... Guilt.

I could not get out of the car fast enough to come in and snuggle my girl. Unfortunately, I would go in every Thursday until August for my Taxol chemotherapy.

There was so much to be grateful for in that moment. I just wished for this summer to go quickly to enjoy being a mom and not a chemotherapy patient. It was such a double-edged sword because as many parents will tell you, time with children goes so quickly.

And it did.

< 169 >

< 170 >

14. STARTING OVER

Beth: For nine months, Jason and I had one goal.

To get Harper here.

> Now she was. When we looked at her, we saw perfection. A beautiful little
> girl with the most beautiful blue eyes. She was eating, not sleeping (at all),
> and if you had not known her backstory, a typical newborn.

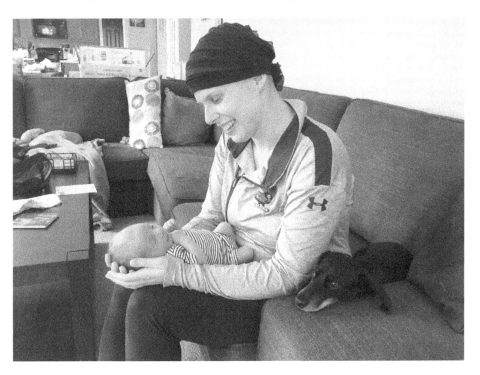

< 171 >

However, with Harper's birth and the ultimate goal fulfilled, the fallout seemed inevitable. The anticipation of her arrival had given us something to look forward to - something to take our minds off of cancer.

That anticipation quickly dissipated, like it had not been there at all.

Instead, it became fear. Fear for Harper's well-being to an extreme. Fear that she would die and all we had been through - the miscarriage, the treatments, the endless appointments, and ultrasounds - would be for naught. That it wouldn't be enough to keep her in our lives.

From the moment Harper's pediatrician told us to keep her from getting sick, I lived in fear. It was like a light switch came on, and I started thinking that basically anything could make Harper sick and die.

Jason: *There is no bigger emotional weight than looking at a tiny baby and realizing that they are 100% dependent on you for their survival. It's terrifying. Especially when you're not entirely sure what you're doing.*

But any of my uncertainty or anxiety paled in comparison to Beth. It's obviously a very different feeling for moms than for dads, especially after the physical act of giving birth, and especially with all of the additional factors that encompassed Beth's pregnancy.

It's probably fair to say all new moms are overwhelmed, but Beth's mindset went beyond that.

Beth: The clinical term is Postpartum Depression that manifests into anxiety. The short term is PPA - Postpartum Anxiety.

It began with handwashing. From the moment Harper came home, Jason and I put bottles of hand sanitizer everywhere. Any time a person tried

< 172 >

to touch Harper, I would ask them to either wash or sanitize their hands. My hands were becoming raw and blistered from the hand washing.

I would get up almost every hour to check Harper in her bassinet because I read about SIDS. I would put her hand on her chest just to make sure she was breathing.

Logically, I knew that Harper had antibodies from me, but at the same time I was terrified that because of the chemotherapy, much of that immunity had been wiped out. Every day, I feared Harper would die. The OB/GYN was right - the feelings that had manifested themselves into insecurity about food during pregnancy were thriving under the guise of Harper getting sick.

These feelings were only exacerbated by the premise of nine more weekly chemotherapy treatments.

This made Harper's first month of life, a time that should have been overflowing with joy, just one more period of challenge and difficulty.

However, there were at least 10 moments each day that we just looked at Harper and just smiled.

During the first week, most of the days, Jason and I followed a set routine:

- Not sleep
- Feed Harper
- Change Harper and/or get pooped on by Harper
- Attempt to sleep when Harper did
- Watch this beautiful little girl take in the world

< 173 >

The first week, we were able to attempt tummy time with Harper because she now had a real belly button.

She hated it. It was not just that she did not like it. Harper screamed bloody murder. I am surprised the neighbors did not come over.

Jason: *It was amazing how this little girl, just days old and not even weighing six pounds, was running things around the house.*

If she was happy, we were happy. If she was unhappy, we were unhappy.

If she wanted to eat, we dropped everything to feed her.

If she soiled a diaper, we dropped everything to change it right away.

It's one thing to know, on an intellectual level, that your life is going to change when you bring home a baby. It's quite another to have it actually happen. It seemed every waking moment and thought were devoted to her. It was not unusual those first few weeks to look at the clock at night, see it was after 10:00 p.m., and realize we hadn't eaten all day. Or showered. Or that we were wearing the same clothes since yesterday.

Beth: Slowly, we began to learn her in those first two weeks. We learned Harper loved skin-to-skin contact. That came from a night that she would not settle down.

Hours into the night, I sat in the beige armchair in our room, threw my shirt off and rocked her against my flat chest. I sang a lullaby in Hebrew... those were the only ones I really knew well.

She fell asleep.

< 174 >

The love we felt during that first month was unbelievable. People made us meals, brought us clothes for Harper, held her so we could do things around the house... our village, once again, came through.

During June, we had so many firsts.

The first time we took Harper out in public. We took her to the community farmer's market, where I saw my students from the previous year. They gushed over Harper with such understanding of what it took to bring her to the world.

The first family nap.... Except I was the only one not napping. Everyone else was, including Percy and Scout. I took a picture to remember the moment.

Within these firsts, June 17th came all too quickly. It marked the end of Jason's paternity leave.

The first time I would be on my own with Harper.

Jason: *It was a very strange feeling to go back to work and immerse myself in that world again. Everything at work took on a different meaning. My perspective had changed so much. On the one hand, nothing seemed quite as important. Project deadlines, returning phone calls, setting up meetings... those obviously paled in comparison to taking care of Harper. But on the other hand, being at the top of my game at work also never seemed more important. After all, I had a family to support now.*

But even as I worked my way through this new dynamic in my mind, I also wondered how Beth would manage taking care of Harper on her own. For the most part, we tag-teamed everything in Harper's first few weeks. No

< 175 >

matter how over your head you seemed in any situation, you knew you could just yell to the other person for help.

Beth: It was amazing and terrifying. However, it also brought the severity of my PPA. After about a week of Jason being back to work, I finally called the high-risk OB nurse who had been my angel for nearly 10 months.

"I need help."

She immediately called the available doctor and got me a prescription for Zoloft. It was the smallest dose they could prescribe. Normally, she said, they would have me in the office for an evaluation. In this case, the nurse knew that the need for help was more immediate.

She also set me up with the counselor through my OB/GYN's practice as well.

It was a tremendous sigh of relief.

Then... finally, Harper met my breast surgeon.

It was a moment we waited eight months for.

The breast surgeon was the first one who looked us in the eyes and told us that we could have this baby.

I had a follow-up appointment towards the end of June, and when the medical secretary called to confirm it, I asked her the question.

"Can I bring Harper with me? Jason just went back to work after his paternity leave."

Her response: "You are not allowed to come if she is not with you."

As I pushed her into the breast center, the moment was surreal. I had sat in that waiting room so many times in the last eight months.

< 176 >

This time felt so different. This time, I was not pregnant. This time, the waiting for Harper was over.

As I walked in, I saw the nurse navigator who had been there since my diagnosis run out with the medical secretary.

They just stared.

"She is beautiful," said the nurse navigator.

No one asked to hold her - I think they sensed my hesitancy, fortunately.

The appointment pertained to the next steps. I was in the midst of my fifth round of Taxol chemotherapy, but soon I would start radiation. With that being a late addition to my treatment plan, I did not have a referral to a doctor in the system.

The breast surgeon seemed pleased with my overall healing on the left side and did a breast exam on the right. However, she kept staring at my head. My short hair - but it was hair.

Finally, she asked.

"Were you blond before?"

I laughed out loud because the oncologist had asked me the same thing the week prior.

This brings to me my other first during this time period.

The first time I had ever been a blond.

< 177 >

My hair quickly began to grow in during my "chemo break" before delivering Harper. That's always a common tidbit you hear from people who went through chemotherapy.

Often, their hair comes back with something different - different color, different texture, different look.

I had very wavy brunette hair prior to chemotherapy. Now, my hair was coming back straight and blond.

Anyone who knew me asked about it upon seeing me. It was pretty interesting, to say the least.

My breast surgeon finished her exam, and then her eyes shifted to Harper, who was sound asleep in her stroller.

I smiled and asked the other seemingly obvious question.

"Do you want to hold her?"

The breast surgeon smiled and made a quick beeline to the sink.

"Uh - YES."

She washed her hands and carefully picked Harper up. She held her close and walked around the tiny examining room, just rocking her.

What a moment. We all had waited for this moment.

This woman kept both Harper and her mama safe for so many months. She cared for us, not just as an incredible surgeon, but as a mother.

The nurse navigator snapped a picture of the three of us as a memento. It was one of the most special moments of my life.

Harper became quite the traveler that week - at least within the Cincinnati area.

< 178 >

The next day, Harper visited Jason's workplace and met his co-workers. Watching Jason's boss, particularly, get so excited about holding her brought us so much joy. It was truly bliss.

Another first for Harper was her first ultrasound because of her kidney. The pediatrician recommended, at her one-week appointment, that Harper have an ultrasound to see if her kidney issue had resolved. Fortunately, there was an outpatient office near our house. I fed Harper prior to the appointment with the hope she would sleep through it.

I was so nervous sitting in that waiting room. I could feel my heart leaping from my chest. It can take weeks for an anti-anxiety drug to work. Sitting in the waiting room made me want to scream.

Germs and sick kids could equate to automatic death for Harper.

After what seemed like forever, the ultrasound tech called us back into this dark, tiny room. I handed her Harper, and that's when I first found out about the magic of Children's Hospital. This tech laid Harper down on her stomach (still sleeping mind you), and completed the test with such love and care. She gently moved Harper's arms and legs into position without even waking her up.

We made an appointment with an urologist to read the results in a few weeks, and until then, we would wait.

Our family had made it through the first month of being a family of three, five chemotherapy treatments, and Jason returning to work. But I would be lying if I said I felt wonderful.

Instead, it felt like a hole, and I was doing everything I could to claw out of it.

< 179 >

< 180 >

15. PARENTING

Beth: As summer rolled on, we continued to give Harper new experiences. After all, that is what maternity leave is for - bonding with your baby.

For the July 4 holiday, Jason and I hosted a few of our friends, some of whom were meeting Harper for the first time.

At the end of July, my best friend from Texas came to visit Harper. We met in Cincinnati in 2009 when I had just moved back to town and commiserated quite a bit during our first years of teaching. Even though she moved to Louisville and then Texas, she was a constant in my life. She had traveled back and forth several times over the last few months to help take care of me. Fittingly, when she arrived, she presented Harper with a onesie that said, "My Auntie in Texas loves me."

Harper and I were active – exploring the zoo, taking walks around the neighborhood, and even enjoying some people watching at the mall.

Yet in the midst of all of this, when I should have been having fun, I was screaming inside. As much as I wanted to enjoy every moment, I struggled to do so.

I just wanted to finish. To be done with chemotherapy.

Taxol was notorious for being cumulative. Each week, I felt worse than the week prior. Exhaustion, joint pain so excruciating that it was painful to

< 181 >

walk, and the beginnings of neuropathy. When I ran my fingers under water, they would go numb. I stopped being able to feel the tips of my fingertips. There was really nothing that could be done for it.

Just get through it.

And once again, my new blond hair began to fall out. Again. Back to headscarves.

It felt like starting over for the umpteenth time.

This was supposed to be the happiest time of our lives - spending this time with Harper. We knew that this would be our first and last time at home with a baby. The baby snuggles were incredible, but the anxiety made it so hard to soak it in.

Jason: *Though we were doing our best to enjoy this time, to live in the moment, it was obvious Beth wasn't able to fully immerse herself because of everything going on.*

Outwardly, we probably looked like any other family with an infant. But to us, everything just felt a bit off, like we couldn't fully relax and live like a "normal" family. Not yet anyway.

Beth: On July 17, I met with the radiation oncologist for the first time. Part of me did not want to meet ANOTHER new doctor. I loved my breast surgeon and oncologist.

And then I met him.

He was awesome.

< 182 >

This appointment was a consultation of what radiation was and why I needed it. He did an unbelievable job explaining it all and even used the dry erase board to demonstrate what radiation did to cancer.

It was like being in the presence of a fellow teacher. Not once did I feel talked down to or demeaned. He truly cared about me understanding each step. In my eyes, he fit in with my two other doctors, whom I held in high regard.

Plus, he was hilarious. He also had a baby at home who was a little bit older than Harper. During this appointment, Harper screamed pretty much the entire time.

"I am used to this," he said. "It's no problem at all."

Although I was absolutely mortified that I could only hear every third word of what he was saying through Harper's screaming, he never once became frustrated. At one point, he held Harper to try to calm her down.

The radiation oncologist explained that when cancer invades the skin, the cells become much more fluid. The cancer is more likely to invade the bloodstream. Chemotherapy starts the process, and then radiation steps in and finishes the job, so to speak.

"We prefer you start within a month of finishing chemotherapy."

The issue was our upcoming trip to Florida. I would need to be available for 30 days straight with no break…but we had already bought our plane tickets. However, he assured me that the vacation would be no problem. He told us to enjoy our trip and confirmed we would schedule my radiation mapping when I got back.

< 183 >

I just wanted to finish radiation, and it had not even started yet.

At the end of July, Harper had her own doctor's appointment - her two-month checkup with the pediatrician. We saw the pediatrician who had taken care of her at her one-week-checkup.

The nurse weighed Harper. Harper ate fine, but she was spitting up a lot at night.

She only gained two pounds.

When the pediatrician walked in, she sat down on her stool. I held Harper in my arms.

"Harper has not gained enough weight until this point," she said in a soft voice.

I immediately started bawling.

This was my fault. I thought we were doing the right thing for her. How could this happen?

"How - could - this - happen?"

"Sometimes, babies just need a little more help. It's just important that we intervene."

I continued to cry. I felt an immense amount of guilt. Maybe we were not meant to be parents if Harper was not gaining weight. How could we let this happen? If I had been able to breastfeed, would this have still been an issue?

The pediatrician made some suggestions in terms of the measurement of formula. As opposed to getting a traditional amount, she wanted us to add an additional half-scoop when making her bottles. Instead of waiting until a four-month checkup, she wanted us to come in at three months to have Harper weighed.

< 184 >

She also explained that Harper was likely spitting up due to the type of formula, but that would cease as her stomach grew. She gave us samples for the sensitive type in that brand.

As we left the office, I called Jason, absolutely inconsolable.

"Of all the problems we could have, Beth, this is one that can be fixed. She will be just fine."

Jason: *Given everything that had happened to our family, I actually wasn't the least bit bothered by the news. I never viewed it as an indictment on our parenting abilities. We were learning how to be parents and as with all new parents, there were a million things we didn't know. It wasn't like we weren't trying – we just needed a little advice, and after all, that's what these appointments were for!*

Beth took it much harder than I did though, feeling as though we were failing as parents already. But I just tried to maintain - and pass on to her - a little perspective. There were parents whose two-month checkups with their infant who received far worse or dire news than this. This was not a life-altering problem. We just needed to add some more food to her bottle and we could fix this quickly.

But I'm not sure that message got through that day. And understandably, as Beth was dealing with a wide range of emotions that I couldn't possibly understand.

Beth: Ultimately, of course, the pediatrician and Jason were correct. Harper quickly started gaining weight, and she was finally on the chart at three months, and then was in the 50% by four months.

< 185 >

It honestly came back to feeling so guilty about what I could not give Harper during this important bonding time. That feeling never fully went away.

Bottom line - I just wanted to finish chemotherapy. Hopefully, at that point, everything would look a little better.

Jason: *It was an odd time for us in the midst of this journey. We were so focused on getting to Harper's birth and making sure she was okay that we didn't think about what would come next. When we were learning how to be parents while Beth still dealt with chemo, and then later, radiation. In some ways, it felt like we could take a breath and relax, while in other ways it felt like we still had so much of the race to finish.*

Getting to Harper's birth had been a monumental milestone for us, but we were quickly learning that the daily challenges were still coming. It wasn't like a movie, where we hit a high point and then the credits roll, with everyone living happily ever after. Instead, we were navigating highs and lows each day, and just trying to figure it out as best we could along the way.

< 186 >

16. LAST CHEMO TREATMENT

Beth: August 1.

The last box to cross off.

After months of sitting in the infusion chair, spending hour after hour watching the bags slowly drain as the minutes dragged on.

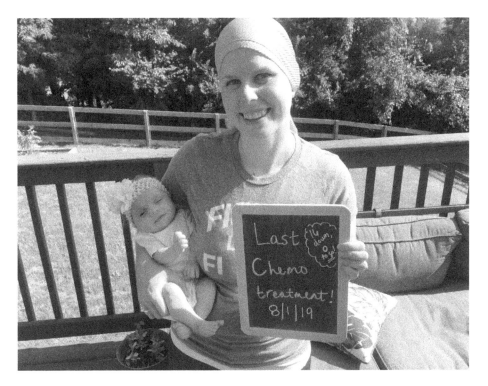

< 187 >

But no more. Today was the day of my last chemotherapy treatment.

Eight months and 16 treatments brought me to this moment.

Even though Harper woke us up two times during the night, I was wide awake even before my alarm. I shook Jason awake. The grin on my face was ridiculously wide.

"Today is the day."

Jason: *The excitement for that day was palpable. Chemo had been such a big focus for her for the last eight months, not only physically, but mentally and emotionally. Between the treatments themselves, the side effects, the dizzying fatigue, the constant doctors' appointments...it had been like an unwanted anchor in our lives for so long.*

It was like waiting for Christmas when you're a little kid and the calendar flips to December. You know the day is getting closer, but the days just can't pass quickly enough.

Except we obviously weren't little kids waiting for Santa and presents. This was a bit bigger. We were counting down the days for an event that would mean Beth got to continue living and see Harper grow up.

Beth: I jumped out of bed and into the shower. I rubbed shampoo into my still very bald head, grasping the baby hairs growing back even so slowly. Never would I have to worry about my hair falling out again.

The plan was that I would go to my appointment at 11:00 a.m., and Jason would bring Harper to the cancer center to meet everyone. It would be the first time that my oncologist would have seen her. After nine months, she could meet the other life she saved.

< 188 >

As I came out of the shower, Harper began cooing for her breakfast. I grabbed a bottle from the fridge and set it in the bottle warmer. As it was finished, I brought the bottle to her and pulled her from her bassinet.

Harper just smiled. It was like she knew today was going to be a great day.

We spent the morning playing and snuggling. Harper had just started to show true smiles, so it was so much fun to just be with her.

I threw on my "Fight Like Fiona" shirt for this significant day... and a pink head scarf to match.

That shirt had come full circle.

I picked out the perfect outfit for Harper - a gray bow and her onesie that Jason gave me for Christmas. It appropriately read, "My mom kicked cancer's butt!"

At 10:15, it was time for me to go. My hands were completely full with treats for the infusion nurses and gifts for my oncologist and nurse navigator. Jason walked me to the car with Harper in tow.

"I should be done by 1, so I'll text you when I am ready."

After I got into my car, I pulled in my "chemo mix" on Spotify for the last time.

The first song was Fight Song by Rachel Platten. My unofficial anthem for the last few months.

I immediately started bawling.

I made it.

Scratch that - we made it.

< 189 >

We made it through that first infusion of blood red toxic liquid being pushed into my veins.

We made it through clumps of hair falling out on my pillow.

We made it through hundreds of doctors' appointments, filled with uncertainty.

We made it.

I walked into the cancer center like so many times before. However, this time was different. This one meant no more chemo.

"You have a huge smile on your face. This is it!" said the receptionist, who already began typing in my information. She was always the friendly face I needed, even on the most difficult days.

As she checked me in, she asked when Harper was coming. The real reason everyone was excited was for Harper's arrival.

I sat in the familiar waiting room, relaxed. Although I knew that in a few short hours, I would likely feel like dirt. It did not matter.

This marked the end of another chapter to this story.

Jason: *It's hard to describe the emotion we felt that day. As I was getting Harper dressed at the house while Beth waited at the hospital, it was hard to keep from smiling.*

We knew, intellectually, that this day was coming; in fact, we had it marked on the calendar for quite a while. But it still felt surreal to look back at where the last few months had taken us, everything that had happened, the emotional roller coaster we had been on.

< 190 >

About eleven months earlier, we received jarring and devastating news. News that was life-changing, and news that for some, can be life-ending. Though we always were optimistic about Beth's plan, the simple truth is that with cancer, there are never any guarantees.

Now, we were getting ready to celebrate her final day of chemo treatment with our beautiful daughter, who we didn't even know was coming when we heard Beth's diagnosis. It truly was incredible.

The versions of Beth and I who sat in that doctor's office the previous September would probably not have believed where they would be by the following August.

Beth: "Beth?"

One of the medical assistants walked me back. We chit-chatted about her boys starting school and football practice.

As I started down in the familiar chair in the exam room, she looked at the computer and broke out in a smile.

"Last one, huh? Are you excited?"

"Yes. Yes, I am."

She checked my vitals and said that the oncologist would be right in.

After a few minutes, there was a knock at the door.

I heard "Hello!" in a familiar voice.

It was my oncologist, and her smile was almost as big as mine.

"This is it!"

< 191 >

We talked about next steps, radiation and still months of targeted treatment to go. However, chemotherapy, we hoped, was forever in the rear-view mirror. I would see her again in three weeks.

"I have something for you."

I handed her the bag, and she lit up. In that moment, all I could think about was how not every story ends like mine. Not all appointments end in gifts and hugs. Some "last" appointments end in very different conversations.

She smiled and said, "Well, can I open it now?"

She pulled out a pullover from Highlands that she could wear to her children's sporting events. I also had tucked in a shirt for her son who was starting his freshman year in a few short weeks.

She came over and gave me a huge hug, and I stuttered to find the right words. How could I? This woman was responsible for both Harper and me being alive.

"Thank you for everything."

She walked me back out to the waiting room, saying she would see me later when Jason and Harper arrived.

It only took a few minutes to hear one of the nurses call my name.

"Beth?"

I came into the now familiar room, but knowing this was the last chemotherapy treatment I would endure made it a little easier. One of my favorite infusion nurses put on my bracelet and asked me the familiar question.

< 192 >

"Birthdate?"

"1/28/87."

I sat down in my infusion chair and ready for me was a warm blanket and Sprite with pretzels. The nurse put the needle into my port and began preparing my premeds. The last IV Benadryl nap was on the horizon.

Then, one of the other nurses came in carrying a bouquet of pink roses.

It was from my in-laws to mark the occasion.

I began to tear up. This was it.

The two hours of premeds and chemotherapy seemed to drag on in anticipation of Jason and Harper's arrival.

Finally, with a half hour left, I texted Jason that I was wrapping up. He said that he and Harper would be on their way.

I came to find out that Harper and Jason had their own adventure prior to meeting me at the infusion center.

Jason: *I was going to be cooking a special, celebratory meal that night and already planned on heading out that morning to get all the ingredients. This would also mark my first trip to a public place with Harper on my own, which turned out to be very memorable, though not in a way I could imagine.*

There were three items I needed to accomplish that day: 1) buy all the food, 2) go home and begin prepping the meal, and 3) get Harper changed into the special onesie Beth picked out for her for that day.

Two out of three isn't bad, I guess.

< 193 >

The grocery store trip seemed uneventful...at first. We had a pretty tight timetable, so I moved quickly throughout the store and grabbed what I needed while Harper cooed and smiled from her car seat nestled tightly in the shopping cart. More than a couple people stopped me to comment on how cute she was, giving me "proud dad" vibes, and foolishly making me believe that taking her out in public was actually pretty easy.

As we stood in the checkout line, I was feeling pretty good about the whole adventure. An older lady behind me smiled at Harper and said she was the "cutest baby she's ever seen."

I smiled as I snuck a peek ahead of us at the man who was finishing paying. We were just a minute or two from getting out of here.

It was at that precise moment an unmistakable sound arose from the shopping cart. I knew it before I even looked down.... Harper had just let loose with a monumental blowout. No need for details, but let's just say nobody around us was doubting what just happened, based on the noise, smell, and yes, even the sight. I did not look back, but I am guessing the older lady behind me was no longer of the belief that Harper was the cutest baby she had ever seen.

But what to do? We were boxed in at the checkout line, next to pay, and I didn't have a clean diaper with me – I had left everything in the car. So, I figured we might as well finish checking out, and then I would deal with everything.

I hustled through paying, then whisked Harper out to the car, where I assessed the full scope of the damage. Her onesie was headed straight in the garbage when we got home – that much was for sure. What I didn't

< 194 >

plan on was the stained, and extremely stinky, car seat. It clearly needed to be washed and I wasn't sure I'd have the time before we had to get to the hospital.

I rushed home, where I stripped Harper down, quickly unloaded the groceries, started marinating the steak, and then set to work on taking out the car seat cover so it could be scrubbed. We were within an hour of needing to leave for the hospital, so using a washing machine and dryer were out of the question. I cleaned everything as best I could be hand, doused it with Febreze, and let it sit outside in the sun until the final minute before we had to leave. Sensing that I was working quickly and trying to accomplish something, Harper made sure to cry and scream almost the entire time, adding even more stress to what had suddenly become a rough morning.

And yes, between scrubbing the seat, trying to calm her down, prepping dinner and making sure I was ready....I forgot to put Harper in her special onesie.

Like I said, two out of three isn't bad.

Beth: Beep! Beep! Beep!

The IV machine indicated I was finished with my last chemotherapy session. That was it. At that moment, I heard the receptionist say, "They're here!"

Grabbing my bag and flowers, I walked out of the infusion suite with two of the nurses whom I became particularly close with.

There was Jason holding Harper... my baby, who was in an outfit that I did not pick out for her.

< 195 >

It did not matter. Each nurse and receptionist took turns holding Harper. The joy in that moment was contagious.

Then, my oncologist and nurse navigator came from around the corner. My oncologist's eyes lit up.

I asked, "Do you want to hold her?"

Her face broke into a tremendous smile and said, "Of course!"

I could feel the hot tears fill my eyes. I watched her cuddle my little girl, rocking her.

This woman worked so hard for seven months to not only treat my cancer but to keep Harper alive. She made decisions for both of us without compromising my care and Harper's safety.

She was the reason we both were there, alive.

And now - they finally could meet in real life. Harper was here and thriving.

After yet another round of passing Harper around to get those incredible baby snuggles, we were on our way home.

At home, more surprises awaited at home. Jason had balloons and matching shirts for Harper and me to celebrate this accomplishment. He also had a special dinner ready.

Another chapter closed. Time slowed and sped in the same movement. With chemotherapy finished, there was preparation for another chapter, radiation.

However, the rest of the month was free - no cancer related appointments and no treatments until the last week of August. Just our family and maternity leave.

< 196 >

It was odd and felt like we had all the time in the world. However, Harper continued to grow. She now finally broke 10 pounds, and one evening during that first week of chemotherapy, we heard the most glorious sound.

Her laugh. We ate hamburgers off the grill one evening, and I propped Harper up on my legs. I stuck my tongue out at her.

The laughs started coming.

"Is that funny?" I asked her.

Harper just laughed.

We sighed in relief and laughed with her. Another milestone crossed off.

Although I would not be starting the school year, I still needed to prepare for my substitute. It would be the first time in 13 years of public school, four years of college, and 11 years of teaching that I would miss the first day, albeit for the best reason ever.

It felt so odd. I had ended the school year early, and now, I was not starting the next school year either.

Strangely enough, once the school year started, I did not even think about it anymore. Things seemed to go well, and I could enjoy the moments I had with our family.

Among the incredible moments was from a wonderful organization in Cincinnati.

A few months earlier, two of my biggest supporters - my nurse navigator and my best friend from high school - saw me absolutely falling apart during the transition from pregnancy to postpartum. Without me knowing, they wanted

< 197 >

to put fun back on my calendar. They nominated me for a gift through the Karen Wellington Foundation.

During one of my chemotherapy infusions, I received an email. I could not have anticipated the impact it would have.

It read: "Spa Day - Karen Wellington Foundation."

The foundation was founded by Kent Wellington who lost his wife to metastatic breast cancer. It provides "gifts of fun" to women living with breast cancer. These gifts include spa days, vacations, and experiences. Initially, Karen's dream, prior to her death, was that when she was cancer-free, their family would provide a vacation to another family dealing with cancer. After her passing, her family continued that legacy.

Jason: *The Karen Wellington Foundation would eventually become a second family for us. It is filled with some of the most incredibly selfless and courageous people you will ever meet.*

We didn't know it at the time, but Beth's spa day was going to open the door for a relationship that would change our lives in a whole new way.

Beth: Inside of the email I received was an invitation to a full spa day with a friend of my choosing.

For 10 months, I had not thought of anything else except cancer and being a mom. Now, I had something to look forward to. Some fun.

23 days after completing chemotherapy, I sat in a different chair.

A pedicure chair.

< 198 >

Instead of tears, I shared laughs with my best friend. My best friend who had been there for me through it all and knew that I needed this.

I was still bald, still sick, but I did not feel miserable.

I felt beautiful.

I felt truly beautiful for the first time in 11 months.

Even with no hair, no eyebrows, and no eyelashes.

This was a turning point for me. I still had radiation and immunotherapy to go - all during my daughter's first year of life.

That day gave me strength to go forward.

August finished just as quickly as it started. One more month of maternity leave prior to heading back to school.

< 199 >

< 200 >

17. RADIATION

Beth: My maternity leave was quickly winding down, and with that would come not only the return to school for the first time in almost five months, but the start of the next phase of my treatment, radiation.

Radiation differs greatly from chemotherapy in the sense of timing. Chemotherapy was in weeks - you would come once a week or once every three weeks. Radiation was thirty days - five days a week for six weeks. The first five weeks would be whole breast radiation. The last week would be a "boost." This was the targeted zapping of my mastectomy scar line.

This all had been a "late addition" to my treatment plan. After a particularly long day the previous March, I received a phone call from my oncologist after seeking a second opinion from the Mayo Clinic (the hospital had a partnership with them).

"They recommended radiation because of the cancer invasion to your skin," she said.

It felt like this moment was far in the future... until we actually started the planning process. The six weeks off most of my treatments (except for immunotherapy) felt like a tease. The Herceptin and Perjeta had few side effects except for a constant runny nose.

"I feel like I need to buy stock in Kleenex," Jason said each time he came back from the grocery store.

< 201 >

That six weeks felt like the ultimate tease. It had been a month of normalcy, and now we were being thrown back into the throes of cancer treatment.

More like catapulted back into it.

Now it would be daily visits to the hospital, not just every few weeks.

However, prior to that, a few steps needed to happen.

First, I would need to go through radiation mapping. This would involve a CT scan to see the proper place that radiation would need to happen. A personalized plan would be created for my case by a physicist, radiation oncologist, and radiation therapist.

Jason: *Much like chemo, radiation was a concept I knew nothing about as it related to cancer treatment. And, perhaps foolishly, I didn't think it sounded nearly as bad as chemo when it had been explained to us initially.*

Maybe that's because we could start to see a finish line at the end of the journey. Maybe it was because we felt like the one of the biggest hurdles had already been cleared because Harper was already here. Or maybe it was because Beth already showed she could handle just about anything that I didn't think this would really faze her.

In fact, I remember hearing the schedule and thinking that one of the biggest challenges was not going to be handling the radiation, but managing the logistics of going to the hospital every single morning before she went to school.

Once again, my ability to be wrong was rearing its ugly head.

< 202 >

Beth: The Edgewood Cancer Center was completely under construction in preparation for a brand new building, so navigating that place was overwhelming, to say the least.

Once again, the mood of the waiting room reflected how I was feeling at that moment. Because it was a different treatment center, I knew no one.

No faces whom I had come to love.

It felt like starting over with cancer yet again. It is amazing how knowing people makes the experience at least a little bit tolerable.

"Birthdate?" the receptionist asked.

"1/28/87," I replied robotically.

I could not believe that I needed to do this - the other ladies knew this information. They still asked, but it felt different coming from them.

Then, I just waited until my name was called. I created a story on Instagram with the checklist.

Surgery ✓
Chemo ✓
Next up... radiation.

It was more to get my mind off of everything.

It didn't.

"Beth Brubaker?"

A medical assistant came over and brought me back into a maze of plastic wrap and the distinct smell of fresh paint.

< 203 >

Finally, we came to a room with a large machine that I was unfamiliar with. I assumed it was the CT machine for mapping. It was a long white board that was on a conveyor belt. That conveyor belt then went into a large opening in the shape of a donut. The machine then scanned you in about 30 seconds.

Then, it spit you out.

There were people coming in and out of the room, wearing masks. It felt so unwelcoming and overwhelming.

As I waited to be loaded into the machine, I began to cry. It was more than tears. I could feel my anxiety creeping into my throat, and that cry turned into a full-on bawling.

The nurse quickly got me a cup of water.

I could barely sputter words.

"H"H-Has this happened here before?"

The nurse nodded.

"Yes, you are not the first one."

It was the emotion of everything spilling out. I am not sure that before that moment I realized I would not be done before my 32nd birthday. Now, it would not be done for months. I think I felt that chemotherapy was the end of a milestone.

It was...but having that time off was a teaser.

It was now months of immunotherapy and a full month of radiation.

< 204 >

However, this, I feel like, is where the battle needed a full-on sprint. But in a moment, I feel like giving up.

I finished my last sip of water and dried my eyes. My breathing was still quite heavy, but I was calm enough to do this.

I put my arms up and listened to the machine catapult me back into the donut. I could feel it whizz around.

Buzz.

I would rather not do this.

Buzz.

What if there is more cancer in my chest?

Buzz.

This sucks. I just want to be home with my daughter.

Then, just like that, it was finished, and they said I could leave.

All night, I kept refreshing MyChart. I wanted to see the scan results - if there were any signs of cancer present.

Finally, I saw on my phone - "You have a new MyChart message."

I quickly scrolled down and saw words - "CT of the chest for radiation therapy planning. No significant abnormalities."

An enormous sigh of relief.

I would complete a "dry run" for radiation on Friday, September 27, 2019. Then, on Monday, September 30, I would start for real. On the same day

< 205 >

that I would return to teaching for the first time in almost five months. My stomach did knots at the thought of that.

One thing that we would have had already tackled is Harper's first daycare experience. Prior to me even becoming pregnant, my co-workers talked about this daycare that served a neighboring school district.

At one point, there were seven teachers at my school with children in this daycare. As one of my colleagues said, "It's no frills, but those ladies love kids."

There was no doubt where Harper would attend daycare.

Because I had a few appointments, I figured it would be an opportunity to do a dry-run for a first day of daycare. We dressed Harper up in a blue romper and lace socks, and then I wrote a first-day sign for her.

I packed her into her pumpkin seat, and when I pulled out of the driveway, I promised myself I would not cry. Harper quickly fell asleep (as she always did), and my mind raced.

This would be the first group of individuals to care for Harper outside of our family. The impact of that weighed on my soul as a mother. So much of me wished I could stay home with Harper. Financially, it was not possible.

Jason: *I suppose I didn't realize how hard daycare would be when we had first started talking about it. Harper obviously needed to be somewhere during the day while we worked and with the recommendations Beth received, it just made sense. Problem solved, right?*

But as the day drew closer, it really sank in for me. Someone else would be in charge of caring for our child. Her well-being was entirely out of our

< 206 >

hands for much of the day. It had always been Beth or I — and usually both of us — working to care for Harper since the day she was born.

Now we would turn her over to someone else, someone we didn't know. Our little girl, who we loved more than anything, would be with strangers throughout the day.

It was a hard concept to get used to.

Beth: I brought Harper into the "Center," as it is affectionately called, and there were older kids sitting at a table together. The day care director, whom I met when I dropped the forms off, guided me to another room with toys more age appropriate for a baby. There were several cribs there too.

I handed both Harper's bottle bag and diaper bag to the director. She put it down, and then the moment came to hand Harper over.

The day care director scooped her up, and held her against her chest. She then just nuzzled her.

That moment gave me an incredible sense of peace. This woman would love Harper as much as Jason and I do. She would be in the best hands. After that day, Harper's return date would be on September 30 as well.

The last week of September gave us a little bit of a reprieve. Jason and I took advantage of my last week of maternity leave and headed to Florida to visit his parents. This would be a last hurrah before all of our lives returned to somewhat normal.

The trip was incredible. We celebrated Harper's four-month birthday and her first time sleeping in a room without us.

< 207 >

Jason: *It wasn't lost on me that the last time we had been in Florida, a couple weeks after Beth's diagnosis, we were dealing with a mountain of unknowns.*

How would Beth make it through surgery?

Would there be a need for treatments beyond surgery?

Would the pregnancy be okay?

Would our baby be impacted by surgery or anything else Beth might need?

Now, we were here again, with our beautiful daughter, and with Beth having overcome every obstacle in her path to date. It was certainly a time to recognize how grateful we were, even when considering all the struggles of the previous year.

Beth: One of the biggest milestones was that Harper went into a pool for the first time.

This almost was one that I missed.

My hair was growing back after the last shave in August. Unfortunately, it looked similar to Harper's - growing back baby fine and in patches. It looked absolutely terrible, and I was embarrassed.

I was still wearing headscarves to cover it up. My hairdresser said she would tackle it upon our return, but it did not help me right now.

For the pool, a friend of mine gave me a sunhat for a baby shower gift. I finally used it for this occasion. I did not want to draw attention to us at this moment.

< 208 >

However, the hat did not fit my head very well. It kept falling off.

When we arrived to the pool, I went back and forth about what I was going to do. Then, Jason got in with Harper, swishing her around the water.

I was not missing this moment.

"Screw this."

The hat came off, and I made it into Harper's first time in the water.

The rest of the vacation was wonderful. We swam, enjoyed beautiful sunsets, laughed, and took advantage of being able to relax, physically and mentally, for a few days.

Jason: *It seemed that each major milestone of this journey had been preceded by a brief time, maybe even just a weekend, where we had been able to catch our breath and take a mental break.*

The first Florida trip right before surgery. The Gatlinburg trip before chemotherapy. Baby showers. Family visits. Summer barbeques.

To me, this wasn't just coincidence or lucky timing. It showed me we definitely were being guided along this journey, that God was still in charge, even when it seemed like we were in the toughest of spots.

Beth: We came home that Thursday - just in time for that dry run for radiation. I would spend my final weekday of maternity leave at the hospital.

The radiation dry-run was just that - a practice round without the actual radiation part.

< 209 >

My radiation treatments would fortunately be at the hospital where I received chemotherapy. Having that familiarity was tremendous.

The radiation therapists, upon my arrival, led me back to a set of rooms I had not seen before. There was a thin hallway leading to the exam room on the left side. Then, on the right side, there was a large, thick door.

A yellow sign graced that door.

"DANGER - RADIATION IN PROGRESS."

Unsurprisingly, that was the room we were heading to. I could feel my palms sweat and my heartbeat quicken.

I paused before going through that door.

The radiation therapist touched my shoulder lovingly to move me forward. By divine intervention, one of the radiation therapists was the mother of two of my former students. It was the beauty of receiving treatment in the community in which you teach. Her touch immediately brought me to somewhat of a place of ease.

"It's okay. Let's go."

The door slowly opened. It reminded me of a secret room in a home in which only a few people have access.

It was strangely soothing. On top of the ceiling were clouds scattered in a bright sky.

Then, the machine.

A radiation machine is like nothing I have ever seen before. I thought the CT scan machine was overwhelming, but it has nothing on a radiation machine.

< 210 >

It is a large machine with a table right in the middle. Above the table is what looks like a camera attached to an arm. That camera will make a large half circle to actually provide the radiation.

The radiation team creates a mold to keep the appropriate body part steady. For me, the mold was a place for me to lie down and put my arms up, leaving my chest exposed.

I took my shirt off and laid on that table in that mold. Once again, the entire hospital had a view of my chest. The radiation therapist left the room, going to the control room next door.

"You are going to have to practice holding your breath for this," she said.

"Why?" I asked.

She explained that by holding your breath during each radiation pass, it essentially moves your heart out of the way to avoid damage from the radiation beams.

Holding your breath?! I could not get over how simple that was.

Then, we practiced. We practiced how much of a breath I needed. We practiced the timing.

When it was over, the radiation therapist gave me a list of dates. It was insane. A long list of endless dates that seemed impossible to do.

Upon arriving home, Jason snatched the list of dates and created another calendar for me to check off dates. He even printed one for school. This one had Mr. T on it.

So many emotions were coming on that next Monday. We would enter a new phase of normalcy... without it actually being normal.

< 211 >

18. WALK

Beth: "Normal" is a very interesting term.

What does that even mean?

> In the span of a summer, our family's lives shifted dramatically. Jason and I became parents with all of the joy and struggle that came with that. I finished one part of my treatments, only to be continuing one set and starting another. I began to look and feel slightly more like myself, thanks to my hair returning, therapy ongoing, and my strength coming back.

It was now time to return to a major part of my life.

Teaching.

The morning of my first radiation treatment would also mark my return to teaching.

I was absolutely terrified.

> For a long time, so much of my identity was wrapped in teaching. I would work hours upon hours on lesson plans and grading. The amount of hours was ridiculous. However, I was rewarded for that through praise and awards. I was a teacher first, and then everything else was second.
>
> Then, my life blew up. They diagnosed me with breast cancer and then I was pregnant. I made it through the entire school year, managing doctors' appointments, chemotherapy treatments, and so many side effects.

< 213 >

I realized quickly that, although I loved teaching, it could not be the priority at that moment.

After spending almost five months as a mother and two years as a wife, I realized that I could never function like I used to.

Entering my classroom filled me with dread, worrying I'd let down my family, students and bosses. What if I could not do it all well?

However, there was no choice in the matter. I would enter my classroom on September 30, 2019 with five classes of students whom I have not met.

The weekend before, my best friend from college came in to see us and take my mind off what was coming. I also had my first haircut to even out my regrowth. I wanted to go to school with no hand scarf and wig. I was going to rock my baby hairs.

Jason: *I knew she was nervous but I also knew she had no reason to be. Much like when she had originally told her students about the diagnosis, I knew she was again giving these kids a lesson much bigger than anything they would learn in their textbooks.*

Seeing her persevere through everything, getting through chemo and surgeries while pregnant, giving birth, and then returning to work, was inspirational. High school students may not remember everything they learned in the classroom – I know I sure don't – but lessons like this would stick with them forever.

Beth: Monday morning came very quickly.

My alarm went off at 5:00 a.m., but I was already up. I tiptoed downstairs to make a cup of coffee and began my typical morning routine... except

< 214 >

the end. The end part involved getting my four-month-old up, changing her diaper, and getting her ready for her first real day of daycare.

I threw on a blue top and checked my radiation bag - tank tops, Aquaphor, and calendula cream. These had been recommended to me to keep the effects of radiation to a minimum.

Before leaving, I made sure all of Harper's bottles were made and in a lunch bag. I wrote an obnoxiously long note with instructions for her daycare teachers. I could feel hot tears in my eyes and my stomach in knots. Giving my girl a squeeze was what I needed in that moment. I kissed Jason goodbye and made my way to the car.

I closed the garage door behind me and instead of music playing in the car, I drove in silence. I just listened to myself breathe. My nerves were shot. They were frayed to no end.

My car arrived at the cancer care center all too quickly. The sun was up and already bright. I grabbed my bag and walked through the automatic doors. I waved at the receptionist, who checked me in.

Chemotherapy was to the right... I was going to the left.

To Radiation.

The waiting room was different. Maybe it was the absence of the fish tank or the lighter color in the room.

It just felt different.

Another gentleman was waiting there when I sat down. He looked about in his mid-sixties. We exchanged looks, and then he went back to his magazine, and I fumbled with my phone.

< 215 >

One of the radiation therapists came out.

"Beth, we are running a little bit behind. It should be just a few minutes."

She said another name, which I assumed was the gentleman's. He got up and went with her.

I just continued to wait.

Finally, it was my turn.

The radiation therapist took me back and went through the process, just like Friday.

Get undressed from the top.

Lie down on the table.

Reach up for the handles.

However, this time, it was for real.

I heard the machine start up and began to move.

"Now Beth, hold your breath."

> The machine moved slowly, beeping every few seconds. The arm passed over my face multiple times. I could feel my lungs screaming for air.

"Let it out."

This repeated three more times.

And that was it.

I slathered Aquaphor on, put on my white tank top, then blue shirt, and off I went to school.

< 216 >

Upon my arrival, I walked into my class, and new faces were there. Those were my sophomore advisory students whom I did not know and would not really meet until after I finished radiation. I would be late to school every morning until the beginning of November.

Then, I had my planning period to breathe. My colleagues came in to say hello and give much needed hugs.

However, though it felt new, it also felt like this was exactly where I needed to be.

My classes came in each period, and I jumped right in.

I started the same way.

"I know that the last eight weeks have been challenging, but I am going to give some grace to you. We are just learning about each other. I hope you return it to me."

Each class had its unique personality, obvious from the beginning.

What was incredible is how the rhythm of teaching came back so naturally. I was happy to be there. I needed that normalcy so desperately... just as I did the year before.

However, at 3:00 p.m., I was out the door to pick up my sweet girl from her first day at daycare.

There was nothing like that first snuggle.

And so the rhythm of normalcy continued.

If normalcy was not sleeping because of a screaming baby, getting burnt to a crisp each morning, working through horrific pain, and crossing off a Mr. T themed calendar for 30 days.

< 217 >

Jason: *Why Mr. T? A couple reasons actually. First, it was such a ridiculous picture of him I knew she couldn't help but smile when she looked at it. And second, because what better image to project unlimited strength than a gigantic human being with arms the size of my waist, wearing a dozen gold chains?*

But, like the "chemo calendar" I made earlier, I think the visual representation of progress was helpful to her. Especially in this case, since it was every single day. The physical and mental effects of radiation would become more prevalent throughout the month, but I think she appreciated being able to mark off the days as she inched closer to the finish line.

Beth: Each day, my skin was in worse and worse shape. Aquaphor and calendula cream were not touching it, especially under my arm. It just kept getting worse - burns oozing and bleeding.

The radiation oncologist managed the symptoms, but this was part of it. Each session meant cancer cells in my skin were burning to a crisp too.

However, mentally, I was losing it. It was becoming emotionally difficult to be there every morning.

Physically, I was to where putting in my prosthesis and bra was excruciating. However, being uneven meant I had to wear a bra and my fake boob.

I just had to suffer through it for my future.

This was not normal... as much as I wanted it to be. Life would never be the normal I knew before.

< 218 >

Jason: *The radiation regiment was grueling for Beth. There's no way I could truly understand the pain she was in as the month wore on. She was an absolute warrior for being able to get through that — no doubt about it.*

Beth: Although each morning of October was mechanical and outright terrible, Jason and I decided to try and do something for breast cancer awareness.

I decided I wanted to do the American Cancer Society's "Making Strides" walk and raise money for the organization. We registered a team for the event.

After a discussion with my friend and colleague for witty names, "Beth's Bosom Buddies" was born. One of my journalism students even helped with the design of the shirt.

With help from our family and friends, we raised almost $5,000 for the American Cancer Society. We also had a small army of friends and family who were joining us on the day of the walk.

The night before, Jason said he needed to run to the store to grab a few things for the walk in the morning. I stayed and graded papers while Harper slept.

About an hour later, I hear the garage door open, and Jason texted me to come out and help with groceries.

Instead of groceries, it was my mother-in-law. She had flown in from Florida to surprise me and take part in the walk.

I cried... she cried. We all were blubbering messes.

< 219 >

Jason: *My mom and I had been planning the surprise trip for a few weeks, and it became harder and harder to keep it a secret as the day of the walk got closer. Getting out of the house alone had been a challenge.*

But seeing Beth's face in the garage that night, a nanosecond before the tears started falling, made it all worth it.

Beth: The next morning, we were in our shirts, Harper in a pink headband, and of course, it was pouring.

However, Judi packed ponchos, and we were off. Even my best friend, pregnant with her first child, was there walking with us.

Upon arrival, I went to the survivor's tent, sponsored by a local sorority. There I picked up a "survivor" sash. However, I did not feel like a survivor yet. That was a term I struggled with, because I wasn't sure when survivorship actually starts. I still felt very much in the throes of it all.

The gun sounded, and we began our walk.

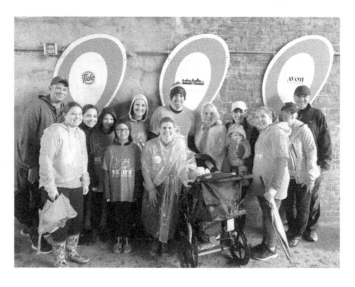

< 220 >

Jason: *As we started down the road, it was hard to not get a little emotional. We were surrounded by thousands of total strangers, yet we all had a common bond. Everyone had their own stories, their own battles, their own physical and emotional scars, their own individual journeys....but we all felt connected in a strange way.*

Seeing all the support systems there, and being there with our support system – it was special. It was a moment when you could forget about all the nonsense of the world and remember what's really important in life – our family and our friends.

Beth: By the end, we were all shivering and soaked (Harper especially), but the morning was incredible. I truly felt loved. I could not stop hugging my friends and family. It was absolutely amazing.

As we approached the finish line, a person was waiting there with a microphone. He was announcing each survivor who crossed the finish line.

He asked each person how long they had been a survivor.

Again, that question.

When it was my turn, he asked me.

"I am still in treatment... I am not there yet."

He announced that as I walked through. Crossing that finish line felt symbolic... just another finish line in this endless race.

I would get the chance to say I was a survivor come Harper's birthday.

May 21, 2020, would be my survivorship day.

< 221 >

< 222 >

19. GIVING THANKS

Beth: It was finally November. More specifically, November brought November 7.

That meant that my Mr. T Radiation calendar would be completely Xed out.

That meant that after 30 days, I would be finished with radiation.

> One of the most difficult parts of going through breast cancer treatment as a young survivor was truly the fact that no one could relate to you. Most women diagnosed with Breast Cancer are much older. The statistics are exactly this - 1 in 8 women will be diagnosed with breast cancer in their lifetime.

1 in 3000 will be diagnosed while pregnant.

Less than 1%.

> At the beginning of my breast cancer journey, I relied heavily on social media in finding others who had or were going through the same experience I was. I yearned for that camaraderie. There was no one in this area who I knew was a young cancer patient, let alone one that was pregnant. The first one I had ever connected to was my friend Terah in D.C. That only happened the previous month.

One of the Facebook groups I found was called "Kick Ass Cancer Mamas."

< 223 >

Every single woman in that group had been diagnosed with breast cancer during pregnancy or within a year postpartum. It was a woman named Leah who had found me in another Facebook group.

Immediately, I felt seen.

A few months prior, the Ohio KACMs wanted to plan an event in Columbus to meet in-person. I fortunately have one of my closest friends in Columbus, who graciously said I could stay with her.

On November 2, I met, in person for the first time, two women who had gone through pregnancy while pregnant. Of all things, we went axe throwing that night.

At first, I was nervous and quiet. The two other women were local and knew each other quite well.

One of them looked at me and smiled.

"Tell us your story."

That broke the ice immediately.

At this point, I was completely raw physically and mentally but felt such a warmth in that moment. My hair was actually showing on my head... with one "chemo curl." Notoriously, hair after chemotherapy comes back VERY curly.

None of that mattered. We bonded in such a way that was indescribable.

One of them had a three-year-old daughter and was considered no evidence of disease. The other woman, who had gone out of her way to

< 224 >

make me feel so comfortable, was Stage IV - chronic, terminal, incurable. The cancer had metastasized to her lung.

We laughed all night. We talked about cancer... but also talked about motherhood. It was such a blessing to talk to women with older children than mine.

I threw a pretty mean axe, and we ended up walking to a taco place that was amazing. The entire night was what I needed after such a challenging summer.

I was ready for the end of the radiation.

That morning, I had butterflies in my stomach. I could not leave the house fast enough. I put Harper into her "My Mommy is a Fighter" onesie from one of our closest friends. In tradition, my "Fight Like Fiona" shirt made an appearance. Although we were rushing around trying to get out the door, Jason made sure to snap a picture with Harper and our chalkboard, just like for chemotherapy.

As I drove to the hospital, all I could think about was the last 30 days.

Thirty days. I have spent 30 mornings in a hospital waiting room. I had sat in the same chair over and over again. It was the worst way to start a day.

My last day, it felt very different from chemotherapy. With chemotherapy, it was a celebration with people who had been with me since I was 20 weeks pregnant. It was with my cancer care family.

I texted Jason as I waited for my last treatment. It felt so quiet in comparison to finishing chemotherapy. I wanted someone to make a big deal about this. It felt like such a milestone because the side effects had

< 225 >

been so tough for me. Whoever said radiation would be a breeze was a damn liar.

Jason: *They told us the effects from radiation would likely end up being cumulative...and they were right. The schedule alone was stressful. Thirty straight days of anything is too much. But the radiation definitely started to take a physical toll as the month went on. She was obviously sore, fatigued, and frustrated at having to start her day this way, every day.*

In many ways, it felt like we were nearing the finish line for this entire journey. And we were. But that didn't mean getting there was going to be easy.

Beth: As I waited for my last treatment, I saw the chemotherapy nurse navigator and one of the cancer care medical assistants. We chatted about babies and church, and how her daughter made a funny old lady laugh in church years ago. It was nice to talk to them to fill the void of quiet.

Then they left. I sat alone.

One of the radiation therapists came and got me. They had really been life savers through the 30 days. There were so many mornings I cried. I cried for being there. I cried because I have cancer. One of them would give me a hug, and the other (as we joked that she tried to kill me during the breath holds) would encourage me and tell me stories about her family, which I appreciated.

The process started like always.

"State your birthdate."

I must have said my birthdate no less than 200 times in the last 14 months.

< 226 >

"1/28/87."

She walked to the radiation room hidden behind a door that clearly marks your fate - "Radiation in progress, do not enter when closed."

I slipped off my shirt. My raw, blistered skin seared in excruciating pain. Anything that touched it felt like a thousand knives mutilating my skin, piece by piece.

However, even with that pain, I could not stop smiling. This was it.

I laid back into my mold with my arms up. The CT machine passed over my chest, as it had done the last 30 days.

It gave me some pause to reflect on this moment.

The whole radiation process differs greatly from chemotherapy. It is very mechanical... routine. You lay on the table every morning - exposed from the waist up. I feel like everyone at the hospital had seen my chest at this point.

Exposed is the only word to describe it. It is cold, white, and very impersonal. You lay there and show the battle scars from this horrific journey. There is no covering up, both metaphorically and actually, what you have been through.

However, in 30 days, I met people along the way - a man who had cancer of the upper lip from smoking. We sat together and talked for 19 of the 30 days. I enjoyed the stories from him about his grandchildren. He loved seeing pictures of Harper.

Then one day, he was gone.

He never finished his radiation on October 28 like he was supposed to.

< 227 >

Then there was another lady. She was really nice. She had breast cancer like me. We chatted every morning.

My thoughts were interrupted by the same words I had heard for 30 days.

"Hold your breath."

Instinctively, I held my breath and closed my eyes. I could feel them watering.

I made it.

After the three cycles, the radiation therapist said I could get dressed. I slathered on Aquaphor and gingerly put my shirt back on.

I took a breath and walked out of the radiation room. There stood the radiation oncology nurse navigator and both radiation therapists. One of them held a certificate.

It read: *"Be it known that Beth Brubaker, having completed the prescribed course of radiation therapy, with a high order of proficiency in the Art and Science of maintaining a cheerful composure while demonstrating high courage, tolerance, determination, is recognized as having earned the respect and admiration of the Radiation Therapy staff and is hereby awarded the certificate of merit (First Class) with all the rights and privileges pertaining thereto."*

Then, I finally was able to ring the bell. The infusion suite did not have a bell, so this was my first opportunity. You are able to ring the bell when you finish treatment. On the plaque connected to the bell, there is a poem that is very prominently displayed. The font is red and sparkly.

< 228 >

It says:

"Ring this bell
Three times well,
Its toll to clearly say
My treatment's done,
This course is run,
And I'm on my way."

My heart pounded as my hand grabbed the bell.

I looked at that bell, and in the background, one of the radiation therapists said, "Did you read the poem?"

I paused again - "Oh yes." That word. I made it through the 30 days.

I rang that bell so hard, and after I screamed, "YAY!" We all clapped, and it was over.

I drove to school, and sitting on my desk was a pastry from one of my co-workers. The day carried on quite normally, but there was a difference.

I would not be at the cancer center that next morning. It would be three weeks before I needed to go back for my regular immunotherapy infusion.

That week, I finally could do a few more "normal" things. I met my student advisory class for the first time - my co-worker and one of my favorite people in the world had been helping me. I finally felt like I was getting to know my advisory students after not meeting them at the beginning of the year.

There was also a very exciting celebration coming up.

< 229 >

My best friend from Columbus, whom I had seen just two weeks ago, was having her baby shower. I was so excited to go through this phase of life with her. Her surprise was due in January 2020.

It would also be Harper's first experience with any sort of gathering that she would actually be awake. I was so excited to show her off to everybody, but most of all I was excited to share this special moment with my friend.

The most that we left, I noticed it. IT was finally making its appearance.

A small, out-of-place curl. A sign of my hair returning (again)... a "chemo curl." This is what I expected after chemotherapy. Curly hair.

Immediately, I Googled some sort of product to help manage it. Yet, it would not cooperate.

The weekend was absolutely perfect. As we spent that Saturday before the party setting up, I just watched Harper sitting in her car seat carrier, taking in every moment.

She was perfection. She was here.

At Harper's sixth month appointment the following, the pediatrician gave us the green light for another momentous occasion.

SOLIDS.

A major causality of my breast cancer journey was not being able to breastfeed. Even though we did not see any sort of lactation consultation in the hospital, and there was no pressure at all to do so, I felt an immense amount of guilt. It was just another experience that breast cancer stole from me as a mother.

< 230 >

I knew for that reason that I wanted to make my own baby food. I had the Pinterest boards, the food processor, and the instant pot in my toolbox.

Jason would walk in on multiple occasions and ask the same question.

"What stinks in here?"

Then, he would light a candle and walk out.

> **Jason:** *Making Harper's baby food was therapeutic for Beth. She was upset that she wasn't able to breastfeed, and this was a way to make that connection with Harper. Like most things in our lives the last year, it wasn't exactly what we envisioned when we had dreamed about kids years earlier.*
>
> *But you adjust. You figure out what you can do within the circumstances and then do the best you can with it.*
>
> *Even if it did make the whole first floor of the house stink....which, being the caring husband I am, I pointed out at every possible opportunity.*

> **Beth:** I was a pureeing machine - sweet potatoes, spinach, peas, and more. I was trying different combinations of everything.
>
> First, we started with baby oatmeal. It was an absolute disaster. Harper screamed and screamed. We were all covered in oatmeal. Percy and Scout, our dogs, did not complain as they licked up said oatmeal.

Finally, Harper did not hate it for a week or two.

Then, it was the moment of truth. Harper would try Mommy's blended sweet potatoes. We sat her in the bouncer and went for it. I shoved the orange goo in her mouth... and Jason filmed the whole thing.

< 231 >

Harper turned in her head, and she looked so confused. It was the first time she had a vegetable like this before. I took the spoon and scooped more into her mouth.

"I don't like them either," said Jason to her reaction.

That was not the face she was making. It was uncertainty.

"I don't think she knows," I said.

Then she looked at me and opened her mouth.

It was a success.

Most of all, it was finally an opportunity for me to nourish my daughter with something I made. It was a tremendous moment of pride and release of some of the intense guilt I felt for not being able to do so earlier.

We could give an immense amount of gratitude on Thanksgiving surrounded by friends, family, and a teething six-month-old for those special moments.

Jason: *It would be a stretch to say that it felt like a normal Thanksgiving. Beth still had treatment left and her cancer journey was not over.*

But there were also times, here and there, when we started to just feel like a normal family. When we felt like any other set of parents dealing with a six-month-old. Trying to balance work and family life, trying to get sleep, and trying to figure out the whole parenting thing. It felt good to be THAT family, even if it was just for a few moments every day. It served, for me anyway, as a reminder of what our end goal was. And that was enough to keep us going.

< 232 >

20. FIGHT LIKE FIONA

Beth: A year ago, I was preparing for a life-altering moment.

I was getting ready to lose a breast at 31 years old.

I was making all the preparations for my students' exam week, and I was trying to calm their fears of not having their teacher there. At this point, they did not know what the complete picture looked like.

Now, I was finished with 75% of my breast cancer treatment and preparing for Harper's first Christmas.

I was preparing for a "life-changing stage." However, it is one that no booklet can prepare you for....survivorship.

The anticipation was different now. It was not a fear of cancer but almost a fear of getting too comfortable.

We were throwing everything at this cancer - surgery, chemotherapy, radiation, and now targeted treatments. What if in a year, two years, 10 years...it was not enough?

Going through cancer treatment is like climbing a ladder - sometimes you go five steps up and sometimes four steps back. Eventually, you come close to the top. You are out of the initial rise - full of bumps and bruises.

< 233 >

The question finally crosses your mind - "Now what? How do I go on living after going through these moments?"

Jason: *When this journey originally started, I hadn't told many people outside of our inner circle. I lean away from over sharing on many subjects, and given that this wasn't exactly easy or fun to talk about, I landed on the side of not saying much. Nobody at work outside of my immediate department was aware. Many of the guys I played basketball with every week had no idea, and even some of my friends were a bit in the dark except for some scant details.*

In some ways it was nice to have a few circles in life where this wasn't the main topic, where there wasn't a constant sympathetic tone as people asked how I was holding up, or how we were doing emotionally. While I appreciated all of that, I also enjoyed some momentary escapes where I could pretend that nothing unusual or dynamic was happening in our lives. Moments where things felt....normal.

But we both figured there would come a time we would have to put ourselves out there a bit. In fact, it was a promise we made to ourselves when we started this journey. Knowing we could hopefully inspire somebody, or give them an emotional boost, overrode our hesitation at putting ourselves out there. We knew it wasn't going to be easy, and Beth was especially worried.

Beth: Every day felt borrowed. What if this was my first and last Christmas with Harper? I felt as though I would not heal. I was still undergoing the Herceptin and Perjeta treatments for my sub-type breast cancer, so I visited the infusion room every three weeks.

< 234 >

However, we were taking steps to be normal. My students would do their typical projects for their AP exam (always a little stressful!). Then Christmas would be spent with Jason's family, and then two days after Christmas, we would be off to Gatlinburg (not before, of course, a Herceptin and Perjeta treatment).

I promised myself that I would attempt to enjoy it.

Jason: *So what does all this have to do with Fiona? For that, we have to go back a bit. A few weeks after Beth's diagnosis, my department surprised me with a gift basket full of goodies for us. I returned to my office after a meeting and encountered a giant basket where my keyboard used to sit. I was so surprised at first that I actually took a step back outside to make sure I was in the right office.*

Food gift certificates, homemade baked goods, blankets, candy, even a bottle of bourbon. It was enough to make me tear up (for the first and hopefully final time!) in the office. To say we were blown away would be a massive understatement.

And though we were unaware at the time, one item in that basket would serve almost a symbolic link from the beginning of our journey to the end. This is where Fiona came in.

Like many people in Cincinnati, Beth became enthralled with Fiona, the baby hippo at the Cincinnati Zoo that was born prematurely in 2017. Given long odds to survive, Fiona showed a fighting spirit from the start, and combined with the loving care of an extremely dedicated zoo staff, she had continued to grow and mature. She became more than a popular animal at the zoo; she became a spirit of hope for many people. The zoo regularly shared videos of her progress, from being bottle-fed to learning to

< 235 >

eat on her own, from testing the water for the first time to swimming happily by her mom.

It was definitely a feel-good story. And naturally Fiona's likeness found its way onto an array of products, from Christmas ornaments to stuffed animals to coffee mugs to shirts. Likewise, most of those items then found their way into our house.

A friend and co-worker, Kim, shared Beth's passion for Fiona. And so, when I found a "Fight Like Fiona" T-shirt in the gift basket, I knew who was responsible. In fact, it was Kim's constant monitoring of new Fiona products, and suggestions about what I should get Beth, that did quite a bit of damage to my wallet!

Beth, of course, loved the shirt. And she wore it for the first time a couple weeks after getting it, as we set off for the hospital for her first surgery. I snapped a picture of her in the shirt to send to Kim and everyone else, and at that point, didn't think much else of it.

Until, that is, Beth's second surgery, when she donned the shirt again before we set off for the hospital. It seemed we found a bit of a good luck charm. The shirt would again make appearances on her final day of chemo before Harper's birth, in the hospital when Harper was born, and on the final day of radiation (as well as plenty of days in between). In fact, Beth's growing belly necessitated the need to get a larger size, just so she always had one available.

Beth: At the beginning of the month, Jason, Harper, and I sat at dinner, and I happened to be wearing my "Fight Like Fiona" shirt. It was the first time since completing radiation in November, and honestly, it was one of the most comfortable shirts I owned.

< 236 >

"We should write a letter to the zoo about this shirt," I said to Jason half-jokingly.

Jason looked at me, surprised, and then vigorously nodded his head.

"You should. Absolutely. [The zoo] would probably love to hear some good news."

In pure Beth fashion, I got busy and forgot about it. This was my busy time of year at work, and honestly, between that, Harper being seven months old, treatments, and chemo brain, I was not thinking clearly at all. Definite tunnel vision.

However, Jason had not forgotten. He ended up writing a two-page letter with photos from the entire journey to Thane Maynard, the executive director of the Cincinnati Zoo. He would not let me read it until it was already sent.

Honestly, a response was not at the forefront of our minds. We had the holidays coming up. Our annual Christmas party. Harper seeing Santa for the first time through Jason's work. She did not realize what was happening and just smiled for the camera.

Jason: *I drafted the letter and dropped it in the mail...and then pretty much forgot about it. A couple of weeks later, I was out of town again for work. After dinner, I got back to my hotel room, logged on my computer and saw a LinkedIn message from someone at the zoo. It was someone in their public relations department, wanting to connect with me over the letter I sent.*

Curious, I provided my cell phone number to her and said I would be happy to talk the next day, when I would have plenty of time while on the road home. I then called Beth, ready to share the interesting news.

But she beat me to it.

< 237 >

"Somebody at the zoo reached out about that letter," she said, her voice a mixture of excitement and anxiety. "They want to do a story on us, and they want to send a reporter to the house."

Talk about unexpected.

Beth: Jason left the decision entirely up to me, but he made the point of saying that this could raise awareness, given the time of year, for the organizations that have helped us.

Although I had been public with our social media pages, this would become much larger than that. This would publicize it for the tri-state region. However, Jason and I made that promise early on that we would help others if we made it on the other side of this. We were now truly testing that promise.

I texted Jason a little later that night.

"Let's do it."

I was admittedly nervous. This was putting a spotlight on our daughter as well. That was not lost on either of us.

A few days later, the reporter reached out to us about setting a day and time. We actually had a connection - her daughter was a student at my school. She was also an award-winning writer, so Jason and I felt confident she would do a great job.

The reporter and the photographer from the newspaper showed up at our house two nights later. I pulled on my "Fight like Fiona" t-shirt with a pink sweater. Harper wore her big pink bow, and Jason held her close.

< 238 >

The questions began, and with each one, I heard my words sputter and fall out of my mouth. I am not sure I was making coherent sentences.

We talked about the shirt and where it came from, and how it was inspiring. Jason showed her the letter, and it was the first time I read it. I could feel the tears in my eyes.

After the interview, the journalist said, "Are there any organizations you would like to highlight that helped you personally? This is the time of year people want to help."

With no hesitation, I said, "Chicks 'n Chucks and the Karen Wellington Foundation." Both had done so much for our family.

The reporter told us that the article would be online in the coming days and published in print on Christmas Day.

Before leaving, the photographer wanted to take a photo to go along with the story. He snapped a few, stopped, and then said, "Let's do one more."

CLICK - CLICK - CLICK.

The photographer looked down and smiled at his camera.

"And that's why you take one more picture."

That picture truly captured our family. The Christmas tree in the background, Harper playing with her feet, us smiling. It was pure joy.

We then waited to see when the article came out.

< 239 >

On December 18, 2019, I received a text from one of my close girlfriends at 6:00 a.m.

"Did you see the article? It's amazing."

Jason and I were both inundated with wonderful texts, social media posts, and messages. The story was doing exactly what we hoped.

Helping other people find joy.

One of the most telling moments came from Jason's work. They posted our story to his firm's social media account, and it was the first time that many of Jason's co-workers knew what was going on (besides us having a baby).

Jason said one of his co-workers, whom he frequently partnered with on projects, popped her head into his office early that morning.

"I had no idea you were going through all of this."

That co-worker got a lesson that everyone is fighting a battle we know nothing about.

Jason: *The day was a bit of a blur, honestly. A lot of co-workers reached out and while there was still some unease that something so personal was now fully out in the public, I also felt optimistic that some good was going to come of this.*

In fact, later that afternoon, somebody pointed out to me that the story had also been shared around Facebook and was receiving dozens upon dozens of comments. One commenter even discussed her recent cancer diagnosis, and that reading our story was inspiring to her as she was starting would what be a difficult journey.

It was exactly the type of impact we hoped it would make.

< 240 >

Beth: A few days later, the reporter called me and asked where, if there was a request, we would like to receive mail or a package. Our preference was the newspaper office, and then from there, it would be forwarded to us.

A week later, we received a package addressed to Harper from the newspaper. Inside, there were two books about Fiona the Hippo directly from the artist and publisher. They invited us to get them signed next time the artist visited the Cincinnati Zoo. It was wonderful.

The momentum of the article carried us into Christmas, which would be Harper's first. At seven months old, she did not understand the meaning of the holiday, but she understood that things were a little bit different.

Jason's parents joined us for Christmas Eve services and preparation for the next morning. One of the best moments was taking Harper's picture in my baby rocking chair next to Santa's cookies and our tree.

I had very few things from my childhood that I kept for my own baby. Things were lost. This chair, however, was one that my grandparents kept, and as I was getting ready to move back to Cincinnati after college, my grandmother sent it back to me.

Many children sat in that chair - a close family friend and both of our nephews.

Now, our daughter. The daughter whom this time last year we were not sure would be here.

Harper was here and smiled so hard at the sight of the twinkling lights and everyone fawning over her.

On Christmas Day, we picked up both the local edition of our newspaper as well as the national one.

< 241 >

There we were on the front cover.

Jason: *Even knowing it was coming out, and even with the reception we had received with the story being posted online, it was still surprising to see our picture, front and center, in the paper. I picked up extra copies to mail to our family members and a couple to save for Harper when she got older.*

Seeing our story continue to spread was humbling, and we just kept hoping that it would help people in some way. We said if it just impacted one person, it was worth it.

Beth: The holidays finished with a trip to Gatlinburg with Jason's mom's side of the family, which was a blast... except for all three kids becoming sick. All were running fevers at various times. Jason also had a terrible bout of food poisoning.

In my head, I was psyching myself up for my next Herceptin and Perjeta treatment three days after Christmas. I was also dealing with horrific skin issues with my treatments.

However, 2020 meant the end of my infusions, and the end of active treatment. The end was finally on the horizon.

< 242 >

21. PERCY

Beth: 2020 brought a new sense of hope to our family

This would be the year that Harper would turn 1 and have made it through the ever important first year of life. 2020 would also bring the last of my breast cancer treatments. We began this journey almost two years ago, and now there was a definite end.

New Year's was so much fun this year and it did not involve me falling asleep on the couch of our friends' house. Although, to my defense, when this happened the previous year, I had just been recovering from my mastectomy.

This year, Harper was all dressed up in her first New Year's onesie, and she even went to bed before the ball drop, allowing us to spend some much-needed time with our friends.

However, even with that sense of hope came another incredibly difficult moment in our house.

Jason: *It seemed that the flip of the calendar unleased a flood of misfortune. 2020 was not yet three days old when my car was rear-ended coming home from work, an accident that led to nearly five weeks of trying to maintain my sanity while working with the other driver's insurance company to get the repairs paid for. (And in the "you-couldn't-make-this-up"*

< 243 >

category, less than 16 hours after I finally got my car back from the repair shop, somebody backed into it in a parking lot).

Eight days after my accident, I witnessed a horrific car accident directly in front of me that totaled two vehicles and sent one driver to the hospital.

We also bought a new water heater in January, an expense we had decidedly not budgeted for, and there was also the deep tissue tear I suffered playing basketball in mid-January, adding on more medical bills.

But all of that paled in comparison to saying goodbye to Percy.

Almost 12 years old, Percy was my black lab that I got less than a month after buying my first house. In fact, one of the primary requirements when searching for that house was a fenced-in yard so I could get a dog. I could live with a small kitchen, bad carpeting, or ugly paint jobs in the bedrooms. But I needed to have a place where my future dog could run around!

And to put it simply, Percy was the best dog anyone could ask for (I recognize that nearly every dog owner says this about their dog, but I think that's fine. It just speaks to the bond that people form with their four-legged friends). But from the start, Percy and I were best buddies. We walked around the neighborhood almost every night, went hiking together on weekends, wrestled and had endless games of fetch, both inside and outside. He had the best demeanor — very calm, very loving, very sweet. He loved to play and had boundless energy, but he also was caring, in the way that only dogs can be.

You can imagine what it was like for me to watch Percy get older and start to suffer from some health problems. There was the sprained joint that had him limping and whimpering for a few days the previous summer. There

< 244 >

was the infected tooth/root that had to be removed in the days after Harper was born. But the most serious was the mass that slowly started forming behind his left eye.

A few rounds of tests and a biopsy revealed that it wasn't, as had been previously diagnosed, cancerous. But without extremely invasive surgery, which wasn't recommended for a dog his age, there was no way of knowing exactly what it was.

Beth: After one such vet visit around this time, our vet dropped the words we inevitably knew were coming but were still hard to fathom.

"Keep an eye on him, but you will know when it is time to take the next step."

Over the Christmas holiday, we had noticed that Percy's energy level had taken a serious nose-dive. He would just migrate from couch to couch in our house. It seemed like eating was painful for him, and he was very lethargic.

He was not himself at all.

Jason: His zest for living was simply gone. He had no interest in playing or even being active. He just looked sad and reached a point where he no longer seemed like Percy.

Beth: Percy was the dog that had unlimited amounts of energy. When Jason and I met, when both Scout, my dachshund and Percy, were a year old, Percy never stopped running. He would zoom around Jason's yard with so much speed. He loved playing with a soccer ball and was a killer Frisbee player.

Most of all, I've never met a dog with his kind of demeanor.

< 245 >

He was loving and incredibly genuine. He would snuggle with you even when you did not want him to do so. When I was off for a week from school during a huge snowstorm in our previous house, I made a fire and laid on the couch, trying to do schoolwork. Percy laid next to me on the chaise lounge and pawed at my hand to pet him.

He loved being scratched behind the ears. Percy had an innate sense of knowing how you were feeling in your soul. Throughout my pregnancy, I would lay the couch, and he would lie next to me, never leaving my side. He was just as excited about a baby as we were. After Harper was born, he would lay next to her as she was sleeping and never bothered her. Percy just wanted to be involved.

His tumor put a stop to all of that. We had watched him stop being Percy before our very eyes.

Jason: *In mid-January, we went to the vet and after a long consultation, we came to the unavoidable conclusion that it was time to put Percy to sleep before he really started to suffer. When you have a pet, you know you'll reach a point someday when they pass away. And if you're lucky, you are able to make that decision before things get too bad for them. But that doesn't mean it doesn't hurt like hell.*

Beth: Jason and I both knew that was coming. He was Jason's dog from the beginning, and he was Jason's best friend. I left all the decisions up to him regarding his care.

With that, Jason decided to come back in a week with Percy to put him to sleep. It would allow us a week to be with him and say our goodbyes.

< 246 >

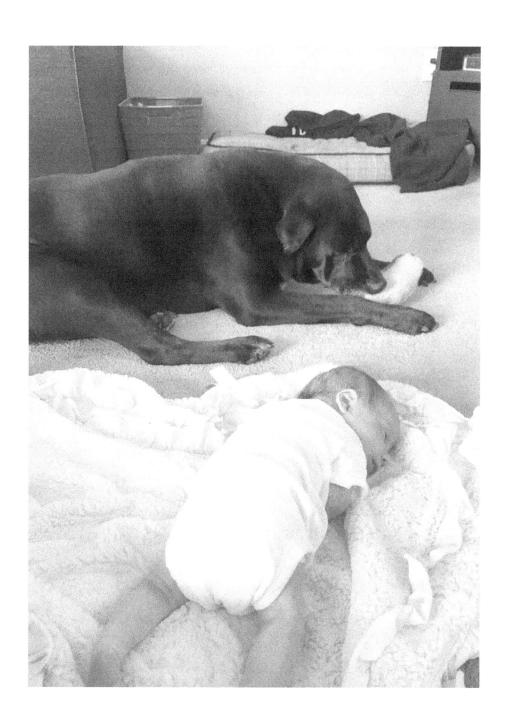

< 247 >

Jason: *Though he didn't have the energy or desire to do much playing, we tried to engage him more over that week, trying to get a few final memories of him. He also ate like a king, enjoying steak, chicken and hamburgers... and more than a few dog treats.*

I dreaded the final day, just because I know how hard it was going to be. With a late afternoon appointment, we had nearly a full day to try to get some last memories. We took him for one final walk around the neighborhood, watching his tail slightly wagging as he made way over the sidewalks. I laid with him on the couch and stroked his head as he slept. Knowing that each passing second was bringing us closer to him no longer being here was hard to grasp.

The time finally arrived, and we clipped his collar on and grabbed the leash to lead him to the car. All I kept thinking about was that we were leaving the house with Percy and we would come home without him. Part of me wished the car ride would last forever.

We arrived to the vet, walked in, took our seats in the lobby, and waited for the vet to call us back. I tried to avoid eye contact with the receptionist or any of the other guests, fearing they would see the tears I was desperately trying to hold back. The vet finally took us to the exam room, where we were given an overview of the procedure. Then, they gave us some privacy to say goodbye.

I asked Beth to leave the room for a second, and I sat down on the floor to get eye level with my buddy. I told him how much I loved him and he responded staring right in my eyes and then laying a wet "kiss" on me by licking my nose. I truly think he knew what was happening. It's said that

< 248 >

animals usually know when it's their time. You'll never convince me that Percy wasn't trying to say goodbye as we sat in that tiny room that day.

Beth came back in and said her goodbyes; we then called the vet back in and he began the procedure. Within about 15 minutes, Percy peacefully passed away as he slept, with both Beth and I sitting right beside him on the floor. It was difficult to do, but we were both determined that he wouldn't be alone when it happened.

As we drove home a little while later, the silence in the car spoke volumes. The rest of that night, and the next few days, seemed to exist in that same familiar fog we experienced so many times over the previous 15 or so months. We were functioning – I went to work the following day, a Friday – but it didn't seem quite real.

There were the reminders at home, starting with the lack of a greeting from Percy when I walked through the door. His favorite toys were still scattered all over the living room. His extra leash hung in the entryway. And Scout was noticeably agitated by Percy's absence. He spent most of the next week or so whimpering and whining while wandering from room to room, trying to find his buddy. It seemed like grief was all around us.

We knew we did the right thing, and there was some solace in knowing Percy was at peace now. But it was tough to know that Harper wouldn't get to grow up and play with him; we always talked about how good Percy would be with kids. All in all, it was just another month in this entire journey that seemed to throw a lot of bad stuff at us. We just couldn't seem to quite get out of the grasp of bad news.

In the big picture, we still recognized how lucky we were. Harper was healthy, and Beth was getting closer to the end of treatment. But Percy's

< 249 >

passing was just another reminder – not that we needed it at this point – of how little control we have over everything. Life changes pretty quickly and rarely goes according to the plans you make.

Percy had been a loyal companion, a great friend, and a member of our family. Saying goodbye was hard, but it turns out 2020 was about to get a whole lot harder.

< 250 >

22.COVID-19

Beth: March brought a lot of excitement in our house after a seemingly difficult start to 2020 - not cancer and chemotherapy difficult but still - more difficult than we anticipated.

March meant I was down to four immunotherapy treatments in my active treatment plan.

Four.

As in less than five. That felt so much closer to being down to less than five.

As in 12 weeks to the title - "Cancer Survivor." A title that I had waited for since September 2018.

March also meant that we were close to celebrating a very special birthday - Harper reaching the all-important one-year mark. We had the party date picked out - Saturday, May 23rd. All of our family would be there, and there would be about 40 more of our closest friends.

Then, life changed. Not just for us... but for everyone.

Jason: By March, we were somewhat finding a routine, busying ourselves with work and parenting, although not in that order. Harper continued to change by the day, developing a feisty and playful personality that made us both anxious to get home every evening and spend time with her. Beth

< 251 >

was counting down the last of her treatments, and things finally felt like they were settling down a bit.

By early March, that last sentence seemed laughable.

Early in January, we all heard about the rapidly spreading coronavirus that originated in China. Truth be told, I barely paid attention to it, and I'm not sure Beth did either. Every few years it seems there was a new disease that was spreading throughout the world and the media always did their part to hype it up and whip people into a frenzy, only to have the whole thing subside in a few weeks.

Beth: I am an avid podcast listener, and since January, The Daily from the New York Times kept mentioning this virus in China. It became known as COVID-19, a type of coronavirus. A coronavirus is a type of virus that usually originates in animals but can spread to people. This one was believed to have originated from a market in the Wuhan Province in China. Common thought is that someone ate a bat and became infected...but who really knew? For a month, this coronavirus spread like wildfire in China and then in Italy.

Words like shutdown, quarantine, and isolation became commonplace on television. The world felt like a scary place.

Then, a few cases popped up in the state of Washington, but it felt like a world away. Most of them were connected to individuals coming back from China. There were so few cases that it felt possible that the virus could be stopped in its tracks.

Jason: But by mid-late February, this story was not only not fading away, it was getting bigger. The number of confirmed cases rapidly expanded, both

< 252 >

in number and geographic reach. Businesses were starting to be disrupted, governments were issuing statements left and right, and stores were having shelves emptied. There was a palpable tension in the air.

At this point, I still thought that this all seemed to be a bit of an overreaction.

Beth: Then, March 11 came.

> **Jason:** A little background - as a sports fanatic, March is one of my favorite months of the year. Conference tournament weekend, capped off by Selection Sunday, and then followed by the NCAA Tournament, is tough to top. College basketball is on all the time, the games have high stakes, and there's just a fun buzz in the air. Even people who don't care about basketball are talking about their brackets. Throw in the fact that the NBA playoff races are tightening up, and baseball spring training is ramping up, and you have a solid 3-4 weeks of sports heaven.
>
> I had admittedly not been as engaged in the college basketball season in 2019-20 as usual. I watched fewer games than ever before and didn't have a real good feel for most of the teams. I guess having an infant at home will do that. But I still was pumped for the tournament. My parents were coming into town for a visit the weekend of Selection Sunday, and it seemed destined to be a great weekend.
>
> However, the first domino fell the Tuesday before this when it was announced that several conferences were planning to conduct their conference tournaments without fans.. They wanted to prevent the gathering of large crowds and potential spreading of COVID-19. It was a giant step that seemed to symbolize the enormity of the situation. There were still plenty of tournaments that were going to be conducted as scheduled, so there was still a hint of "I think they're overreacting" to

< 253 >

conversations. In fact, several NBA teams stated that they planned to disregard suggestions to conduct games without fans, as did baseball teams with regard to spring training games.

But on Wednesday, things escalated quickly. The afternoon saw the NCAA announce that they were planning to conduct tournament games without fans, a decision which was then echoed by most of the major conferences for their conference tournament. A short while later, the conferences began cancelling tournaments altogether.

As sports fans all over the country, including the thousands who traveled to see their teams play in conference tournaments, were starting to process this information, the NBA announced that they planned to conduct games without fans for the foreseeable future. Outside of the sports world, schools and businesses were closing and the sense of panic was increasing.

It was amidst this backdrop that Beth and I sat in our living room on Wednesday night, talking about how surreal it all seemed.

Beth: March 11 is our wedding anniversary. We had gone out to a local distillery the weekend before, and since it was a Wednesday night, we spent the night sipping a glass of bourbon and just relaxing. Harper went down quickly, and we were settling in to watch an NBA game on television.

As Jason was flipping through the channels, he was also scrolling through Twitter.

He stopped and said one word.

"WOW."

I sat up a little straighter.

"What's going on?"

< 254 >

Jason just looked stunned. That rarely happened.

"Apparently Rita Wilson and Tom Hanks caught COVID-19 in Australia."

> **Jason:** *Just a few minutes later, as we tried to digest the Tom Hanks news, I saw a report that a couple players for the Jazz were now being tested for COVID-19, and shortly after that, it was revealed that All-Star center Rudy Gobert had actually tested positive. Four minutes – four minutes! – later, the NBA announced they were suspending the season indefinitely.*
>
> *Talk about a shock. In the span of 48 hours, we had gone from thinking that a couple conference commissioners overreacted by canceling their tournament to watching the biggest basketball league on the planet shut down.*

Beth: A stunning turn of events.

> What had started as a somewhat normal Wednesday evening had turned into the fastest changing news cycle since September 11. Jason and I were frantically texting and scrolling through our phones, trying to get more information.
>
> That night, the world changed forever. There was before March 11, 2020 and after. The world, in the span of one day, looked entirely different.

> **Jason:** *The dominos kept falling. Thursday, the NCAA announced they were canceling the men's and women's championships, thus giving us a March with no basketball. It was unprecedented. The rest of the sports world quickly followed suit, as the NHL suspended play, baseball suspended spring training and pushed back the start of the regular season, the PGA suspended play and delayed the start of the Masters. It seemed every hour there was a new cancellation.*

< 255 >

And it resulted in one of the strangest periods I can ever recall, because there were literally no sports on TV. None. No scores to check in the morning, no game to have on in the background. Nothing. Arguably the best sports month of the year was wiped clean.

Beth: School that Thursday was unlike anything I had ever experienced. We sat in a place of limbo. We were in a place of fear.

The NCAA canceled all post-season tournaments that morning.

I remember sitting at my desk during lunch and thinking about the prospect of actually being in school during all of this.

Ten minutes later, at 12:46 p.m., we received an email from our superintendent. She had just gotten off the governor's superintendent call and wrote the following:

"The governor, upon advice of numerous experts, has advised several measures to try to contain the virus, including limiting visitors to nursing homes, canceling large gatherings (such as church services), and discouraging international and cruise travel. These experts are also concerned that if the virus spreads quickly, our healthcare services will not have enough equipment, gear, supplies and people to meet the patient needs.

By trying to mitigate the disease, stop it from spreading by practicing "social distancing," we would have a chance for our healthcare system to catch up, as well as slow down the outbreak. To that end, today, the Governor advised that schools should be prepared to close (with a 72-hour warning) so Monday would be the earliest that this would occur.

< 256 >

State universities have already announced closures and moving to online learning."

Jason: *This was no longer a disease that had originated thousands of miles away and likely wasn't going to impact me or anyone I knew. Now it was a very real threat and had already started to impact our lives.*

In the coming days, I would find out that a close friend's parents had both been diagnosed, and another close friend's wife had to be isolated as she displayed some symptoms. While this was going on, more and more business and schools were shutting down as everyone scrambled to try to stop it from spreading.

Beth: My phone blew up with texts right after the governor's announcement.

"How are we going to do this?"

"What about childcare?"

"How will this look?"

"It will only be two weeks."

There was no focus for the rest of the day. Teachers were scrambling to figure out next steps. Our tech-savvy students were getting information from parents and sending it to others.

My editor-in-chief of our publications program was already working on an article with all the information needed for students, faculty, and parents.

My brain physically was not computing any of it.

Jason: *It seemed that the whole world was just coming to a screeching halt. And worse, there still didn't seem to be any real answers. There*

< 257 >

was no vaccine, testing was still inadequate, and the only advice experts could really give the general population was to stay home and wash your hands often.

Meanwhile, we watched as Italy and other countries were struggling to keep up with the rapid spread. Death totals across the world climbed. You didn't want to give into the panic and fear, but nobody really knew what to do.

Beth: Leaving school on that Thursday, there was a feeling of impending doom. We knew what was coming now. School was going to shut down to do these days called "Non-Traditional Instruction."

While I was in the car with Harper after picking her up from daycare, I listened to the local NPR station for the Ohio Governor's COVID-19 update. Being in a tri-state area, we can hear news from Ohio and Indiana, which in moments like this, can be helpful. At the press conference, he had his public health specialist there. He talked about things like testing and nursing home shutdowns.

Then he said it.

"All in-person instruction at K-12 Public and Private Schools will cease for two weeks beginning on March 16, 2020."

That's when I knew that the announcement from our governor was inevitable.

About 25 minutes later, it happened.

We would close to slow the spread for two weeks.

< 258 >

Jason: *On the one hand, you obviously wanted to be cautious and safe. We had an infant at home, not to mention Beth being just a couple months away from her final cancer treatment. Either one of them getting a virus, especially one with so many unknown factors swirling around it, would be devastating.*

But on the other hand...how long was this going to last? Surely, we weren't going to be working from home longer than a couple of weeks, right? After all – it's 2020! We're at the absolute peak of medical knowledge and technology. No way this was going to be something we are worrying about for that long.

In my infinite wisdom, I predicted that within a few weeks, this whole thing would pretty much "blow over" and we'd be back to normal by the time we got into summer. I just could not conceive of a virus that could shut down everything in 2020. We were too smart, too advanced for that, right?

Beth: That weekend, Jason's parents were coming to visit us. We had a wonderful weekend with them. Harper started crawling for the first time. She had been trying to for months and finally did it, just a couple hours before they arrived at our house.

For dinner on Friday night, we went to a local pizza place with part of Jason's extended family. It was wonderful. Several of them had not met Harper, and it brought everyone such joy. Harper enjoyed pizza for the first time, much to Jason and his pop's happiness.

It was the last normal weekend we had in 2020.

The next day, everything was different. Fear had settled in. People moved away from one another. If someone coughed, things went quiet.

< 259 >

Jason's parents had decided to drive straight back to Florida on Monday. They would not risk staying at a hotel and bringing something back with them.

We went to dinner one last time together, and the restaurant was packed. One last hurrah until the unknown.

I could feel my anxiety boiling... the same feeling I would get when Harper was a baby. Stifling fear.

Jason: *Selfishly, I figured this summer was owed to us after what we'd been through. Beth would be cancer-free, Harper would be one and able to enjoy summer activities more. We were going to embrace it all.*

Summer cookouts with friends, afternoons at the pool, evening walks to get ice cream, going to Reds games. Life was finally going to be normal again, and no virus was going to take that away from us.

Wrong again.

< 260 >

23. QUARANTINE

Beth: Reaching April 1 brought the start of my "Spring Break." I use that term lightly because there was no break in sight. It became apparent that life would not be returning to normal anytime soon.

The first two weeks of COVID-19 lockdown had been tolerable. I attempted teaching online schooling with a 10-month-old, although most of the time I felt like I was failing. Jason juggled trying to work from home with our whole family constantly in the background. We joked that many of Jason's WebEx calls had me walking back and forth or Harper crying nearby.

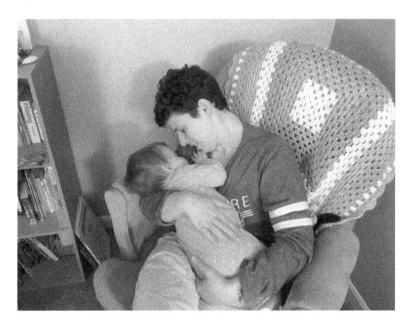

< 261 >

Spring Break brought much of the same except I did not have to go through the routine of posting assignments, chasing down students through email, calling parents to try to figure out why a student was not returning said messages or emails, and managing our actual family.

It was a moment to breathe during a time that was suffocating. After Harper was born, I could imagine myself as a stay-at-home mom. Quarantine proved very quickly that it was a terrible idea. I needed to work.

Jason: *In some respects, the quarantine was beneficial for us. With Beth and I both working from home, we were able to spend more time with Harper than in normal daily circumstances. We were there when she began to crawl, which soon led to pulling up on furniture, which led to getting the confidence to stand by herself for a few seconds, which then led to taking some unassisted steps just days after her first birthday.*

After weeks of babbling, we finally heard her first words, and we watched her proudly test how loud she could screech when she wanted to get our attention. We saw her personality continue to develop into a fun-loving, slightly mischievous little girl who knew exactly how to get what she wanted from her parents.

Chances are, had we been at work and had she been at daycare, we would have missed some of these milestones. So we were grateful for quarantine in that aspect.

But in pretty much every other way, quarantine was abysmal. Sure, we did what we could to liven things up. Zoom calls with our friends. Setting up a "bourbon tour" around our house. Walks around the neighborhood. Letting Harper explore the yard, walk on grass, and touch flowers for the first time.

< 262 >

We even did an Easter Egg hunt in our basement with Harper (who enjoyed shaking them more than finding them).

But it all just felt off to me. People are not designed to stay locked up, away from friends and family. It's just not right.

Beth: In early April, after much uncertainty, I had received a phone call for St. Elizabeth Cancer Care in Edgewood. My oncologist made the call to have my care transferred to Edgewood to ensure I could finish my last three Herceptin and Perjeta treatments on time. That was a major concern, and honestly, it was crushing to think that it was possible I would not finish on Harper's birthday.

That milestone got me through each infusion.

My oncologist knew that and made it happen.

I was able to start my spring break with a tremendous weight lifted off my shoulders. Harper and I would continue our routine of three-mile walks each day and playing at home. The time together would be joyous.

Jason: *Meanwhile, as we tried to just stay focused on our lives and getting Beth to the finish line, the world around us seemed to be crumbling. Businesses were being closed and industries were getting hammered. Employees were being furloughed or laid off. People were literally getting into fistfights at the store over toilet paper and cleaning supplies. It seemed like the entire world had gone mad.*

It felt like the only way to stay sane was to insulate ourselves, taking advantage of time with Harper and burying ourselves in work.

< 263 >

Beth: At this point, I was in my second year of advising our publications program at my school. My Journalism students (7 strong that year) were handling the unknown. There was no playbook for how to complete a yearbook during a global pandemic when we could not collaborate.

A plan was conceived over a Teams call with our yearbook representative. The theme of the yearbook was "The Anatomy of a Bluebird." There was no better show of what that meant than figuring out how this yearbook would look.

We were going to finish it - all 232 pages. We were going to finish it with the hope that we would return to school, and it would be fine.

However, at the same time, that uncertainty was wearing me down.

Would we return to school after Spring Break? How would we finish the yearbook if we did not? When would the lockdown end?

On April 2, 2020, we listened to the Governor's daily address, and heard the news that we would extend the school closures until May 1. Soon after, our assistant superintendent emailed us to share that "we anticipate a return to campus on May 4."

We could only hope.

Everywhere you looked, the strain was becoming evident.

Jason: *Perhaps to cope, people everywhere started referring to this as the "new normal." You couldn't turn on the TV or have a video chat with someone where that phrase didn't come up.*

But no matter how many times I heard it, I still cringed. This was not normal, and I wasn't going to pretend otherwise. I wasn't going to spend

< 264 >

the rest of my life treating everyone I walked by as if they had an infectious disease. I wasn't going to be fearful to leave my house. I wasn't going to settle for human interaction through a computer screen. That's just not how we are supposed to live.

So I refused to accept those weeks as anything other than an aberration, a struggle to get through so we could return to actual normal.

Beth: However, one of the best moments of this month came in the form of a car ride over Facebook messenger.

It was my fellow breastie's (yes – we use that term to describe fellow survivors!) last day of chemotherapy. She endured everything I had thus far - pregnancy, chemotherapy before delivery, delivery, and then more chemotherapy. One of the unfortunate parts of the pandemic is that no one could be in person with her to celebrate.

Her husband and I had the idea of making her a video of her closest friends and family wishing her congratulations and sending love to her. So many of her family and friends contributed, and it was a bright spot putting it together for her.

We decided we would let her watch it while she was in the car driving to her last treatment.

I called her at 6:30 in the morning, and needless to say, she was confused.

"What's going on?" she asked.

We explained that although we could not be there physically, she deserved to be celebrated.

< 265 >

The entire car ride turned us all into emotional messes. Watching her reaction to all these people made the awfulness of quarantine dissipate for a precious amount of time. She would not stop thanking us, but honestly, it was a gift for us to do for her.

We hoped to actually meet in person for Harper's birthday party in May, but again, there was so much uncertainty at that point. No one knew what the next week would look like, let alone a month from now.

Jason: *It was pretty clear by this point that our plans for a grand celebration were going to have to change. Between limits on large gatherings and restrictive travel in some parts of the country, not to mention a general level of fear among many people, the timing just wasn't right for a party.*

The fact that Beth's last day of treatment was scheduled for Harper's first birthday wasn't lost on us, and we believed it was more than a mere coincidence. It seemed like a storybook ending to this crazy journey. We had been so excited to mark the occasion with everyone who helped us along the way. But it just wasn't meant to be, and so, once again, we had to pivot.

And even as we were coming to grips with that, bad news just continued to come.

Beth: On April 28, 2020, we received an email about a faculty meeting. I was the middle of meeting some of my students on Microsoft Teams, and I would hop on as quickly as I could. My students and I wrapped up, and I transferred to the next call. The principal was wrapping up, but he asked if I could stay on the call.

He began with "I am so sorry, Beth..."

< 266 >

He informed me that one of my students was killed in a car accident earlier that morning. My student had been driving when the car crashed – he and another young man died, with two others in the car injured.

I felt like that wind had been knocked out of me. I screamed and sobbed. This young man is one whom I had spoken with a few weeks earlier.

On that phone call, I scolded him about not attending our class meetings or completing assignments. He was a genuine young man with a great sense of humor. He had a great deal of unrealized potential. This student was in my class of 12 - an incredibly tight-knit group.

We could not gather to mourn for him and the other student. We could not hold a vigil and be together. Instead, we sat in our houses alone, unable to truly grieve for these young lives lost.

Our district asked us to leave our outdoor lights on that night to honor these two young men. I took a picture to remember that sadness and isolation in that moment. It encompassed what COVID-19 was doing to us - isolating us from one another.

Jason: *It's awful for any young person to lose their lives – it's something I always struggle to wrap my head around. But to have it happen under these circumstances, when kids and teachers were isolated from each other and couldn't be there to comfort each other in the most tragic of moments, only made it that much worse.*

Even though I never knew the student personally, I was still left speechless that morning as Beth told me the news. There's simply no words that can make something like that make sense.

< 267 >

It just reinforced to us – again – the need to appreciate every day because things can change in the blink of an eye.

That meant we had to figure out a way to make the most of this time, focusing on the positives instead of dwelling on what we couldn't do. That included celebrating the final steps of Beth's journey as we inched closer to her final treatment, even if it wasn't going to happen in the way we initially imagined

Beth: Not long after that, I did my first video visit with a physician - the nurse practitioner from Cancer Care - prior to my infusion the day after. We chatted for a few minutes about how weird it was to be doing a doctor's visit as a videoconference.

Then, she began talking about the "lasts" - my last appointment and last infusion.

"You have not stopped grinning since we started this conversation," she said.

"That's because we are finally talking about the end."

Finally.

I would go to this infusion tomorrow, and then there would be one left on the MyChart calendar.

I was 22 days away from the end. After 18 months, we were down to days.

Finally.

< 268 >

24. DONE

Beth: This is not what May 2020 was supposed to be.

At school, it was supposed to be filled with the grind of AP Testing, the chatter of upcoming summer vacations, the final touches of the yearbook, and the excitement of graduation. It was supposed to be a "normal" end-of-the-year after a trying one the year before.

At home, it was supposed to be preparation for incredible moments - Harper's first birthday, meeting our friends from Washington, D.C., and the last of my immunotherapy treatments. We planned, initially, to have a giant celebration to commemorate the occasion.

Then, COVID-19.

AP Testing moved entirely online. Summer vacations were canceled. Graduation would not take place in our performing arts center.

Our big celebration - postponed. Friends and family coming in - gone. A month that we waited and prayed for, essentially for the last 24 months, looked so different from the original picture in my head.

When May rolled around, I spent time grieving that. However, with the effort of so many, there was light during such a somber time.

< 269 >

Our school administration stepped in and did the best they could for each student, especially our seniors. The teachers in our building delivered cookies and signs to our seniors, signifying the graduation event. I had the privilege of delivering a sign to one of my colleagues and closest friends' daughters.

To see her face light up at a sign in her yard filled my heart with joy. It was some of the first true joy in a long time. I could feel a bit of that "normal" season creeping into my soul.

Then, Mother's Day. Jason and Harper showered me with love that day. Honestly, the greatest gift was to see Harper crawl. Two years earlier, we were faced with the unknowns - the unknown of our nephew's future and of our own future child.

Here we all were. Griffin, now almost two years old, was thriving. Harper, finishing her first year, kept us laughing constantly. We had survived.

I waited patiently for May 21. Harper's birthday and my last treatment. I could feel that immense joy bubbling over in my heart.

Jason: *Even without the big party we planned on, we still had celebrating to do. Beth was locked in on doing as much as possible for Harper that day, including scheduling a family photographer to come to the house, ordering a cake for her to smash, and setting up a Zoom video call with all our friends and family so they could join us, at least virtually, on the special day.*

What she was not thinking about was how we were going to mark the day for her. We had celebrated some special milestones along the way, but this was huge. From the day she was first diagnosed, we wanted nothing

< 270 >

more than to get to this day. Finishing treatment. Walking out of the hospital healthy. Knowing that she stared down a potentially fatal illness, emerging victorious. A hug and a "way to go" just wasn't going to cut it.

Fortunately, although planning ahead isn't necessarily my strong suit, I worked on ideas for months. The pandemic presented some additional challenges, but I was determined to make this day special, regardless of what it took.

I ordered some special gifts, including a Survivor key chain and coffee mug (Beth is addicted to coffee and has no fewer than 50 mugs in our cabinet). When the pandemic closed tattoo parlors and eliminated the idea of me surprising her by getting the pink breast cancer ribbon tattooed on my wrist (an idea we'd discussed), I pivoted and ordered a slate of temporary tattoos, just to show her what the real one would look like. I worked with some friends to order a limited release bottle of bourbon that we could open that night. I even had matching shirts for us – with mine reading "I Wear Pink for my Wife" and Harper's reading "I Wear Pink for my Momma."

But the centerpiece of the day was the video.

For the last eight or so months, I worked on a special video montage to commemorate this journey. Filled with pictures of us that dated back to the bourbon cruise just two days after her diagnosis, I tried to capture the entire journey. There were pictures in the hospital during chemo treatments, celebrating the holidays with family, and fun events along the way – from our trip to Florida to a Sunday at a Bengals game to an afternoon in Lexington where we toured the UK basketball practice facility. I had pictures of Harper just moments after birth, dozens of pictures of her being held by friends and family, and dozens of our first year with Harper.

< 271 >

Visiting the pumpkin patch. Playing with the dogs. Sporting a Halloween costume. Visiting the zoo. Grinning in her high chair while most of her dinner covered her face, clothes and the table. All in all, I had well over 100 pictures in the video, which was set to music and included some slides of inspirational quotes.

I had gone through almost a dozen songs before finally settling on four that worked the best with the pictures. I spent over a hundred hours editing and reviewing the video to make sure it was perfect. But about a month before the big day, I still wasn't quite happy with it. There was something missing.

From the start, I knew I wanted to include "Fight Song," since it's one of Beth's favorite songs and it just strikes the right tone. But in my video, it didn't seem to match with any of the pictures I included. I needed something else.

Then...inspiration. As luck would have it, a couple months earlier, Beth worked with a friend's husband to put together a short video for his wife's last day of chemo. They worked to capture pictures and videos of friends and family, each with inspirational and congratulatory messages for her as she marked this milestone in her journey. Watching it, and watching her reaction to it, sealed the deal. The final piece just clicked into place.

Beth: Those few weeks of waiting did not go without reminders that there was so much sadness in the world.

May 18, 2020, was the first day I was allowed in my classroom since March. They gave us 15 minutes to grab what we needed. They staggered us, so no one else was there.

< 272 >

There was a deafening silence on the 2nd floor hallway, a place that typically is one of the busiest paths in our school.

It was dark. Rain audibly splattered on the roof.

I shut my classroom door behind me and started to cry. The sadness was suffocating.

Finally, May 21 arrived. I stayed up until 12:29 a.m. in order to kiss my girl and tell her Happy Birthday. I just stared at her in disbelief, overjoyed that she was here and healthy.

I could barely sleep that night. The anxious joy pulsated in my veins.

A year ago today, Harper made her arrival, and we breathed a deep sigh of relief.

"Are you sleeping?" I kept asking Jason.

"Yes..." from his side of the bed.

I was up by 5:30 a.m. I kept going through the list for the day.

Get Harper's birthday outfits ready.
Pick up donuts.
Confirm with the photographer.
Go to treatment.
Pick up smash cake.
Get home.
Get dressed.
Pictures.
Zoom.

< 273 >

When I finally woke up, I checked my phone and saw I had a video from my in-laws. They talked about the pinnacle of such a journey and their pride and love for me.

My mother-in-law ended it with a simple reminder.

"Today is also your day. Enjoy every moment."

She knew that, as a mom, my focus would be on Harper's birthday.

I made breakfast and tried to distract myself by dancing with Harper and reciting what needed to be done.

Then, a knock came at the door.

It was my wonderful best friend from high school. She had champagne and flowers in hand.

"I am so proud of you and did not want to miss this moment."

Here came the tears... again.

Soon, it was time to go. I pulled on a pink shirt that a friend had made me for this occasion. It had been sitting in a bag for a few weeks. I decided to retire my "Fight Like Fiona" shirt for this day.

It read: *"Proud wife, mother, teacher and finally, breast cancer survivor."*

When she gave it to me, she slipped in a surprise - a matching one for Harper.

< 274 >

Jason took our pictures with my chalkboard. For each milestone, that chalkboard was a constant.

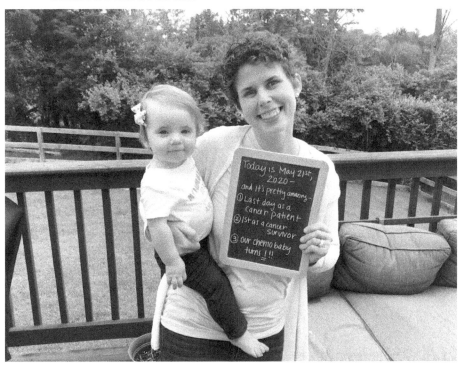

It said:
Today is pretty amazing.
Last day as a cancer patient.
First day as a cancer survivor.
And our chemo baby turns 1.

With that, Jason, Harper, and I got into the car and drove to the hospital. We stopped on the way to grab donuts from our favorite place for the medical staff. Then, off we went.

It was the longest drive in a long time. It may have just been the excitement building.

< 275 >

When we arrived, Jason told me to text him when I was finished. Because of COVID-19, I could not actually go into the building without calling first. Then I would have to wait until they called me back to let me in.

It took about a half hour. Harper, in her car seat, was less than pleased. Finally, the phone rang. It was my turn.

Jason: *Because Harper and I were not allowed in the hospital with her, we had to find a way to occupy ourselves for an hour or so. We drove to get a coffee, but first stopped to change into our new pink shirts, which I hid in my car the night before.*

Beth: I grabbed my mask and walked into the cancer center. The receptionist greeted me.

"Name and date of birth?"

"Beth Brubaker - 1/28/87."

She handed me a paper mask and led me through plastic tarps and the sounds of construction into the infusion suite. I would wait there until the oncologist was ready to see me. A nurse greeted me at the entrance, and she led me to my infusion chair. In exchange, I gave her the donuts.

"These are the best," I told her.

It was an isolated corner, and honestly, I was glad for it. No one would see me cry.

After about twenty minutes, the medical assistant, whom I recognized from my original cancer center, led me back to an exam room.

Quickly, my oncologist came in, masked up and distanced, and remarked, "Today is definitely a good day!"

< 276 >

She did her exam and talked about follow-ups in the future.

I could tell she was smiling under her mask.

"I would give you a hug, but…"

COVID.

I could feel the tears coming. I handed her a card.

"There are no words that I could possibly say to thank you. Thank you for everything."

> We both got up, and she led me back to the infusion suite. I sat down and checked my phone. There were a few messages from some of my infusion nurses from the original cancer center who were working in the other building.
>
> They wanted to come and see me. I was so touched. Although this was not what I envisioned my last treatment to look like, I felt so loved.
>
> The nurse hooked my port up and gave me my Tylenol. We would then wait for my medications.
>
> And then two of my original infusion nurses walked in. I started to cry. They congratulated me and told me how proud of me they were. They could not stay long, but it meant so much to me. They have so many patients, but both of them took the time to see me.

A few minutes later, my last Herceptin and Perjeta bags arrived.

For the last time, the nurse asked me: "Name and date of birth?"

I could not stop crying.

"Beth Brubaker, 1/28/87."

< 277 >

It would be thirty minutes from start to finish of my infusion. I saw my oncologist pop her head in again to get a donut from the box I brought. She waved.

I sat there anxiously, waiting for a familiar sound.

BEEP - BEEP - BEEP.

That meant the bags were empty. For the last time, my infusion bags ran dry.

Just like that, I was a cancer survivor.

I immediately texted Jason.

"All done!"

I waited for the nurse to unhook my bags from my port. Then it was over. Done.

I could not get out of the hospital fast enough. Upon me walking out, I saw Jason's car. I threw my arms in the air. It was a sweet victory.

Jason: *After returning to the hospital parking lot, Harper and I had essentially tailgated as we would have for a football game while we waited for Beth. I played some music, gave her a snack, and we may have even danced a little during breaks in the drizzling rain. And yes, we drew some strange looks from others in the parking lot.*

Beth: on got out and opened the door for me. He gave me a huge hug and kiss. Then, I noticed his shirt.

"I Wear Pink for my Wife."

Then, as I climbed in the car, I saw Harper's onesie - also pink for Mama.

< 278 >

As we drove away, Jason told me there were more surprises coming at home. I reminded him that we had a lot to do before the photographer came.

"It's your day too."

Jason: *We drove home where we started cleaning the house in anticipation of the photographer. Once we got Harper down for a quick nap, I brought everything out. When it came time for the video, I just handed her a box of Kleenexes and we huddled up on the couch in our sitting room to watch it together. By this point, I had watched it through no fewer than 40 times, but because I was so excited for her to see it, it almost felt like I was watching it for the first time.*

I think we made it two slides in before the tears came! And full disclosure, I wasn't far behind. It was received exactly as I had hoped. We laughed at some of the goofy pictures of Harper, wiped away tears at some of the chemo pictures, and by the time the first notes of "Fight Song" came on, she was basically a waterfall.

Beth: Pictures from the last two years scrolled on the screen. Some of the best and worst moments in the last two years.

I was bawling.

Then, pictures and videos from our friends and family started popping up with well wishes.

"How did you do this?" I asked Jason in between tears.

It was absolutely beautiful.

I gave Jason the biggest hug. For a few moments, there was no isolation to be had.

< 279 >

Jason: *She was blown away by all the people who contributed to it, and she was thrilled to know that we essentially had a documentary of this entire journey to show Harper one day when she's old enough to understand. To some people, it may have just been a 12-minute video full of pictures. But to us, it showed the highs and lows of what we had been through, the emotions that swung back and forth each day.*

It was basically the story of our life – the good, the bad and everything in between. And watching it put us right back in many of those moments – sitting in the chemo suite, celebrating baby showers, spending the first night with Harper in the hospital, learning how to be a parent. Each of those pictures carried special meaning for us.

Beth: Not long after the video finished playing, our doorbell rang. Flowers from my best friend from college.

The love just continued to flow... but then, it was Mom time. I got Harper dressed and put her down for a nap. I began getting the house ready for the photographer.

About two hours later, our wonderful photographer showed up for Harper's 1-year pictures and Zoom smash cake party.

I am not sure if the photography gods were shining down on us, but Harper was perfect. She laughed and smiled. We thought she loved the flash of the camera. Every picture was fabulous.

Then, at 5:00 p.m. we turned on Zoom and put Harper in her high chair. I sat the pink cake in front of her. Harper had not eaten cake before, but you would never know. After I stuck her fist in, and she tried that sugar, she went to town.

< 280 >

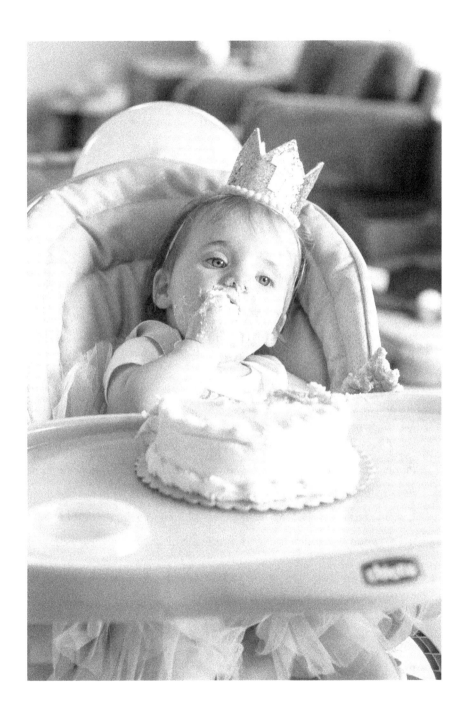

< 281 >

Over 30 of our friends and family showed up on Zoom to watch our 1-year-old eat cake. Our tribe, who had continuously showed up for two years, was there again.

Harper looked so happy. She would have eaten the entire cake if we had not taken it from her.

Our photographer snapped her last picture... and it was done.

Harper's first birthday - via Zoom - was a success.

Jason made a fabulous dinner, and afterwards, we put Harper down for bed. We celebrated the day with bourbon and music.

Jason: *Even though the day wasn't quite like we had imagined it would be months earlier, in some ways it may have been even more meaningful. It was almost like a microcosm of this entire journey - we adapted to circumstances out of our control, kept a positive attitude and made the best out of a less-than-ideal situation.*

All in all, that day gave me a lot to think about as my head hit the pillow that night. When we started this journey, our goal was to simply get to this day — with Harper healthy and Beth being cancer-free. And we had done it. It wasn't easy and it wasn't anything we wanted to go through. But here we were — done. We made it. It was a surreal feeling, just because we looked forward to this day for so long and now it was over.

Beth: For a few weeks prior, I had tried writing a letter for Harper for this occasion.

I couldn't find the words. I was frustrated about it.

Before bed that night, I took a shower... and the words just came to me. It was divine intervention after struggling for weeks. I jumped out of

< 282 >

the shower, grabbed my robe and my laptop. I got into bed and began furiously typing.

"What are you doing?" asked Jason.

"I think I needed to live through the day to write this."

It took 15 minutes to write my letter.

I read it to Jason, and I could see tears in his eyes. He kissed me again.

Jason turned off the light.

"This was a good day."

I rolled over and looked at him.

"It was the best day ever."

< 283 >

< 284 >

25. MOVING ON

Beth: The previous day, we had celebrated the end of a strange, difficult, remarkable, and incredible chapter of our lives.

I wrote the foreword to this book late that night after the words came to me in the shower, long after the festivities of the day. I fell asleep that night with the feeling that someone had lifted a weight off our shoulders.

Within days, it was soon replaced with the weight of a 10,000 pound boulder.

While undergoing cancer treatment, there is a tremendous safety net. Doctors, nurses, and therapists are constantly watching over you. People check every inch of your body parts and blood to ensure that the monster will stay at bay.

Then, at that last appointment, you get a hug (which I did not get, by the way - thanks COVID-19), a "hooray, you are done!" and then sent off on your merry way to live your life. There is an unsaid expectation (unintentionally but still there) that life gets to return to "normal."

About three days after ending treatment, Jason, Harper, and I sat on our deck, grilling out for dinner. Now 1-year-old Harper was prancing around the deck, squealing in glee and chasing Scout.

All of a sudden, I began to cry.

< 285 >

More like bawling.

I could see Jason was caught off guard.

"What's going on?"

The weight of that boulder was crushing my shoulders.

"What do we do now?" I sobbed.

> No one gave us the guidebook of how to navigate life after cancer. In total, one or both of us attended over 100 doctors' appointments in 18 months. We spent five days in the hospital between a lumpectomy, mastectomy, and then Harper's delivery. I had 30 mornings at Cancer Care for daily radiation treatments and 30 various types of infusions between chemotherapy and immunotherapy.

And just like that, it stopped.

Jason said some of the most impactful words I ever heard.

"Beth, now you get to live. Actually live."

> **Jason:** *Whenever I've heard about people who overcome extraordinary circumstances or adversity, I've always wondered how they found the mental and emotional strength to keep going each day. How do they resolve themselves to keep moving forward? Where does that strength come from? Don't they ever just want to give up?*
>
> *It was a little over a year into our journey that it dawned on me... people may be asking some of these same questions about us, and more specifically, about Beth. Because when you look at everything in hindsight, it is overwhelming to think about everything that occurred.*

< 286 >

We found that the truth is when you're in the midst of it, you're just doing what you have to do in that moment, in that day, to get to the next one. You try to stay in the moment and handle what's right in front of you. It's only later, once you reflect on everything, that you think "Wow! How did we do that?"

But though Beth's last day of treatment marked a finish line for us, it wasn't THE finish line. We still had plenty of life ahead of us. But how do you move forward from something like this?

On the one hand, we craved normalcy after all the craziness, stress, fear, and anxiety that essentially governed us since 2018. But on the other, we weren't the same people that started that journey. Things had changed and we wouldn't ever look at things the same way again.

And, understandably, things were much more complex for Beth. It wasn't as easy as just "moving on." This was always going to be a part of her life.

Beth: The bouts of fear and anxiety over the last three years have receded some, but they're never fully gone. In that time, I have watched friends and acquaintances have initial diagnoses of cancer, and some be re-diagnosed with local recurrence and, unfortunately, with Stage IV breast cancer. There is not a week that goes by that I don't wonder if I will be here to see Harper graduate from high school, get married, and start a family.

The best analogy I can give is that it feels like there will always be that gun with a finger on the trigger. Some are fortunate not to receive that second shot in their lifetimes... others not so much. I pray I am on the right side of that trigger.

< 287 >

My oncologist and other doctors say that my risk of recurrence is about 5-6%. I took some extreme measures in lowering that even more by doing a prophylactic mastectomy on my non-cancer side. In June 2020, my breast surgeon sent me for my first mammogram since my initial diagnostic one, and it was gut-wrenching. Listening to the machines whisper and move made me want to puke in the middle of the room. I could not imagine doing that every six months for the rest of my life.

Although my breast surgeon and oncologist assured me it was unnecessary, they understood and supported my reasoning for doing it. It has been two and a half years since that final surgery, and I have not regretted it for a moment. It gave me an immense peace of mind.

Each doctor has now "released" me to annual appointments, so although I see each of them once a year, I will still see someone every 3-4 months for the foreseeable future.

Peace of mind yet again.

Jason, Harper, and I have tried to make the worst experience of our lives into something that can positively impact others in our situation. Through the Karen Wellington Foundation, the same organization that gifted me that ever-important spa day 23 days after finishing chemotherapy, we started a fund in Harper's name.

The Harper Jaye Brubaker Living FUNd targets young mothers living with breast cancer who have young children. The goal is to put fun back on their calendar, allowing them to enjoy life as a human being and not as a breast cancer patient.

< 288 >

The generosity of our family, friends and co-workers in supporting this has been overwhelming. Since 2021, we have been blessed to be able to give multiple gifts to families in our area, ranging from spa days to vacations to annual zoo passes. More importantly, we have built relationships with these families, and they have blessed our lives so much.

It is a lonely place to not only be a family dealing with breast cancer, but to be dealing with it all so young. We never wanted another family to have that feeling like we did.

Jason: *It is not hyperbole to suggest that being affiliated with KWF, and starting the Harper Jaye Brubaker Living FUNd, changed our lives. The ability to help people and brighten their day has been incredible for us. There's a true sense of purpose that wasn't always present for us before this journey.*

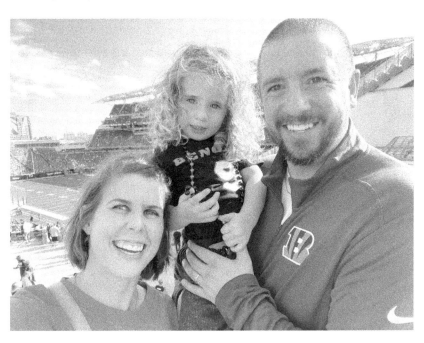

< 289 >

Beth: Our family has almost moved on from this chapter, writing new ones as we go. During the process of writing this book, we celebrated our fifth wedding anniversary with a special trip. We watched Harper grow into a blossoming toddler who is now wrapping up her first year of preschool. And we have made hundreds of memories as a family, from simple days at the local playground to family vacations. We even have added a couple of new four-legged friends to our household, ensuring that while it may never be quiet, we are always surrounded by the best kind of chaos.

The remnants of this experience are still a part of the fabric of our family and forever will be. However, as other breast cancer survivors told me early on, the feeling of losing a sense of self is not forever.

I hope that when Harper reads this story for the first time, she is shocked... not because of the story itself but because her life did not revolve around it. We wanted her childhood to be beyond cancer.

Although we will never completely move on, I believe that we have and will - as Jason said so directly that day - live.

< 290 >

THANK YOU

When we first discussed the idea of writing a book to capture this journey, we had no idea what it might entail. We didn't recognize how difficult it would be to relive moments that caused so much pain, or to revisit feelings that we never fully reconciled at the time. But overriding all of that was the obligation we felt....the obligation to try to support or inspire others who may be on a similar journey. The obligation we have to Harper, so she can know her story.

There are hundreds of people we need to thank for their support, both throughout this journey and throughout the process of writing this book. Though we figured out pretty early on that there was no way we could ever repay people for what they did for us, we hope that everyone knows how much they lifted us, helped us, guided us, inspired us, and helped us get to this point.

To our family and friends: We have been beyond blessed to have an incredible support system of family and friends throughout this. We never took it for granted how lucky we were to have people always willing to step up for us. To pray. Send cards and flowers. Bring meals. Give a hug. Cry with us. Make us laugh. Help around the house. And sometimes, just to sit and talk. It cannot be overstated how much that support meant to us at every step. We are eternally grateful for each and every one of you.

To the doctors and nurses: A simple "thank you" is far too inadequate to express our gratitude to, and admiration for, all of the doctors, nurses and

< 291 >

health care professionals who took this journey with us. Their knowledge and skill were beyond anything we could ever imagine; yet it was their compassion, empathy and genuine kindness that took it to another level. We knew we were in good hands from the first day and we are so fortunate to have had you in our lives. You all are truly heroes in every sense of the word.

To The Karen Wellington Foundation, Pink Ribbon Girls and Chicks-n-Chucks: There are dozens of organizations, charities and foundations out there that offer support for breast cancer patients and survivors. All of them do incredible work. But these three in particular are special to us. Their support lifted our spirits at a time when we needed it most, and we are extremely grateful for all they did for us....and all they do for others. We strongly encourage anyone to donate to these organizations, or others that may be close to your heart, so they can continue to lift others the way they lifted us.

That's why documenting this story was so important for us. We felt we had a duty to so many people. Not only to thank them for their support, but to pay it forward. And if this story is able to impact someone's life, then we'll feel like we've repaid at least a small fraction of what's been given to us.

Finally, Harper, thank you for being a bright light for us. This is truly for you.

< 292 >